Ieva Tolmane
Baiba Rozentale
Raimonds Simanis

Factors Influencing Chronic Hepatitis C Treatment Results

AF138640

Ieva Tolmane
Baiba Rozentale
Raimonds Simanis

Factors Influencing Chronic Hepatitis C Treatment Results

LAP LAMBERT Academic Publishing

Impressum / Imprint

Bibliografische Information der Deutschen Nationalbibliothek: Die Deutsche Nationalbibliothek verzeichnet diese Publikation in der Deutschen Nationalbibliografie; detaillierte bibliografische Daten sind im Internet über http://dnb.d-nb.de abrufbar.
Alle in diesem Buch genannten Marken und Produktnamen unterliegen warenzeichen-, marken- oder patentrechtlichem Schutz bzw. sind Warenzeichen oder eingetragene Warenzeichen der jeweiligen Inhaber. Die Wiedergabe von Marken, Produktnamen, Gebrauchsnamen, Handelsnamen, Warenbezeichnungen u.s.w. in diesem Werk berechtigt auch ohne besondere Kennzeichnung nicht zu der Annahme, dass solche Namen im Sinne der Warenzeichen- und Markenschutzgesetzgebung als frei zu betrachten wären und daher von jedermann benutzt werden dürften.

Bibliographic information published by the Deutsche Nationalbibliothek: The Deutsche Nationalbibliothek lists this publication in the Deutsche Nationalbibliografie; detailed bibliographic data are available in the Internet at http://dnb.d-nb.de.
Any brand names and product names mentioned in this book are subject to trademark, brand or patent protection and are trademarks or registered trademarks of their respective holders. The use of brand names, product names, common names, trade names, product descriptions etc. even without a particular marking in this works is in no way to be construed to mean that such names may be regarded as unrestricted in respect of trademark and brand protection legislation and could thus be used by anyone.

Coverbild / Cover image: www.ingimage.com

Verlag / Publisher:
LAP LAMBERT Academic Publishing
ist ein Imprint der / is a trademark of
OmniScriptum GmbH & Co. KG
Heinrich-Böcking-Str. 6-8, 66121 Saarbrücken, Deutschland / Germany
Email: info@lap-publishing.com

Herstellung: siehe letzte Seite /
Printed at: see last page
ISBN: 978-3-659-48497-1

Zugl. / Approved by: Riga, Riga Stradins university, Diss., 2012

Factors influencing chronic viral hepatitis C treatment results

Table of contents

Abbreviations

a – regression constant

ALAT – alaninaminotransferase

ANA – antinuclear antibodies

ANOVA – ANalysis Of VAriance

Anti-HCV – antibodies against hepatitis C virus

b – regression coefficient

BMI – bone mass index

CC – interleukin 28B gene CC genotype

CI – confidence interval

CT – interleukin 28B gene CT genotype

e – Euler's number = 2.71828

ELISA – enzyme linked immunosorbent assay

Exp (B) – coefficient e^B or OR – odds ratio

F – Fisher's exact test

GGT – gamma glutamyltranspeptidase

gt – hepatitis C virus genotype

HAI – histological activity index

HBs antigen – superficial antigen of hepatitis B virus

χ^2 test – Chi-squared test

HCC – hepatocellular carcinoma

HCV – hepatitis C virus

HCV-RNA – hepatitis C virus ribonuclein acid

HIV – human immunodeficiency virus

HOMA-IR – homeostasis model assessment of insulin resistance

IFN – alpha interferon

LIC – Riga East University Hospital, hospital „ Infectology center of Latvia"

LR – Republic of Latvia

N or n – number

NABs – neutralizing antibodies to human interferon alpha

Non-CC – interleukin 28B gene CT, TC and TT genotypes

p – probability, p-value

PEG IFN – pegylated interferon alpha

PCR – polymerase chain reaction

RBV - ribavirin

r_s – Spearman's correlation coefficient

R^2 – determination coefficient

SD – standard deviation

SE, S.E – standard error of mean

Sig. – significance

SVR – sustained viral response

SPSS – Statistical Package of the Social Science

TC – interleukin 28B gene TC genotype

TSH – thyroid stimulating hormone

TT – interleukin 28B gene TT genotype

ULN – upper limit of normal

VHC – viral hepatitis C

VHB – viral hepatitis B

z – equation of regression

Wald – Wald's criterion

x – values of independent variables

Topicality of research

Due to its distribution and clinical course, chronic viral hepatitis C has become one of the most common infectious diseases in the world. At present the number of the infected in the world is about 170 million, but in Europe it exceeds 9 million. The incidence of chronic viral hepatitis C in Latvia is relatively high. The antibody prevalence is 2.4%, HCV-RNA prevalence is 1.7%, it means that in Latvia there might be almost 40 000 chronic hepatitis C patients.

Hepatitis C viral infection in population has been found quite recently. The virus was discovered only in 1989 when its genome was identified. An opinion prevails that patients' getting infected started faster at the beginning of the 90ties of the past century (donors' blood was not tested) and is still going on due to the lack of vaccine. Chronic viral hepatitis C itself cannot essentially affect the patients' quality of life, however, about 20% of patients are known to develop liver cirrhosis within 10-20 years. Besides, it is impossible to say how long the patient has been infected, as well as whose disease is going to progress to develop cirrhosis and hepatocellular carcinoma (HCC). Since about 20 years have passed from the first diagnosed wave of infection, liver cirrhosis and hepatocellular carcinoma rate at present and in the nearest years is going to grow in the whole world.

When undergoing treatment, 54-63% patients can get rid of hepatitis C virus. Various factors are known to determine and affect the outcome of treatment. First of all, these are the patient's own factors and co-morbidities – age, sex, race, genetic factors, obesity, insulin resistance, diabetes mellitus, HIV infection, smoking, alcohol consumption, each individual's body reaction by developing neutralizing antibodies against alpha interferon, consequently, reducing its effectiveness, secondly, viral factors – genotype, viral load, thirdly, morphological changes before the therapy – fatty liver, degree of fibrosis, activity of inflammation, cirrhosis.

It is, therefore, important to find any factor influencing the treatment result and to correct it, as far as possible, prior to starting the therapy, in order to achieve maximum good therapeutic result.

Novelty of research

During the study there were found the factors influencing the result of chronic VHC treatment. On the basis of these factors, a treatment prognosis model for chronic viral hepatitis C was developed. The information obtained in the study can be used as the foundation for making important decisions when treating chronic VHC patients to improve the therapy result.

Aim of research

The aim of the study was to determine and analyze the factors influencing chronic viral hepatitis C treatment results in order to predict the possibility of SVR.

Objectives of research

1. To analyze the patient's factors (age, weight, BMI, smoking, alcohol consumption, co-morbidities, genetic factors) and the changes of analyses (insulin resistance, cholesterol level, neutralizing antibodies) in connection with the therapeutic effect.
2. To assess viral factors (genotype, viral load) as the indices affecting the treatment result.
3. To analyze morphological changes prior to undertaking the treatment.
4. To determine IL28B gene polymorphism in Latvia and its relation to the treatment result.
5. To develop the treatment prognosis model of chronic viral hepatitis C and to prepare recommendations for the practicing physicians in order to improve the treatment results of chronic VHC.

Hypotheses of research

1. The patient's factors (age, BMI, IL28B genotype), liver functions, changes in metabolic and immunologic indices (GGT, insulin resistance, formation of neutralizing antibodies), morphological changes (degree of fibrosis, HAI), virus genotype and load affect chronic viral hepatitis C treatment result in Latvia in the same way as in other countries.
2. Finding out the factors influencing chronic VHC treatment result, one could predict the possibility of treatment, developing the treatment prognosis model.

Material and methods

Study groups

299 chronic viral hepatitis C patients were included in the study, who had attended LIC out-patient department in the period from 2009 till 2011. The diagnosis of chronic VHC was confirmed performing HCV-RNA test by PCR method. All patients were white race individuals, their average age was 38 years, males – 165 (55%), females – 134 (45%). Previously hepatitis C treatment was received by 34 patients (11.4%) being treated by various medicines – recombinant alpha IFN in monotherapy or in combination with RBV, or pegilated IFN in combination with RBV. Within this study 223 (74%) patients received pegilated interferon alpha 2a 180 µg/week, 71 (23.7%) patients received pegilated interferon alpha 2b 1.5 µg/kg/week in combination with ribavirin 800 – 1200 mg/day, 2 patients received interferon alpha 2a 180 µg/week in monotherapy, 1 patient received multiferon in combination with ribavirin, 2 patients did not undertake hepatitis C therapy.

From all 299 patients 140 (46.8%) responded to hepatitis C therapy, 124 (41.5%) – did not respond, 30 (10%) interrupted the therapy (24 – arbitrary, 3 – due to side effects, 3 – due to financial conditions), 2 – did not start therapy, 3 – have not yet accomplished therapy at the moment of processing of the results (Picture 1.).

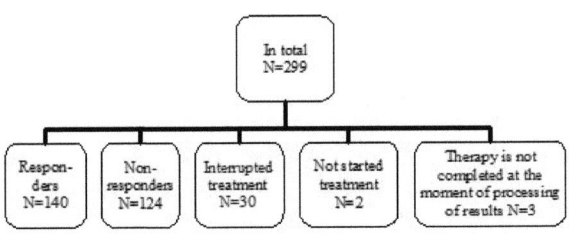

Picture 1. Distribution of patients under study

In order to make the analysis of the factors influencing results of chronic VHC treatment, 2 patients' groups under study were organized (Picture 2.).

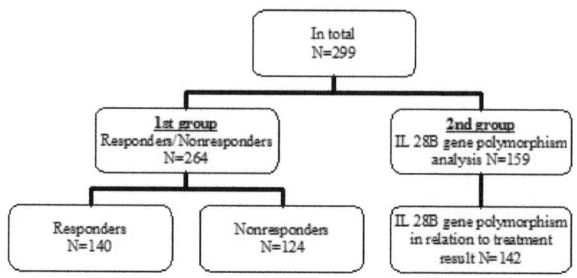

Picture 2. Patients' distribution into study groups

1st group – in order to analyze the factors influencing the treatment results, from all 299 patients under study there were selected 264 with chronic VHC who:

✓ Have received standard treatment with pegilated interferon and ribavirin,

✓ Have not interrupted the therapy arbitrarily,

✓ Have completed the treatment course and have been followed up untill 24 weeks after the end of treatment in order to assess the treatment result.

From all patients of this group 140 (53%) were males and 124 (47%) were females. There prevaled HCV 1st genotype – in 185 patients (70%), 2nd or 3rd genotype was seen in 79 (30%) patients. The mean age was 38 years. From the moment of making the diagnosis till starting the treatment there have passed on average 2.2 years (0.1 – 13.5). All these group patients were divided into subgroups depending on the treatment result:

1. Responders – patients, who have responded to therapy (N=140, 53%) – have reached SVR – HCV-RNA – negative at the end of therapy and 24 weeks after completing of therapy,

2. Nonresponders – (N=124, 47%) – have not responded to therapy, have not achieved SVR:

✓ Null response (N=51) – in 1st genotype patients there is not achieved a hunderedfold HCV-RNA viral load reduction within 12 treatment weeks, the treatment is interrupted, considering that it is going to be ineffective,

✓ Partial response (N=34) – is at least a hundredfold HCV-RNA viral load reduction within 12 treatment weeks, but at the end of treatment HCV-RNA – positive.

✓ Relapse (N=39) – after the treatment HCV-RNA is negative, but 24 weeks after completion of the treatment – positive.

Patient distribution is seen in Table 1.

Table 1.

Patient distribution in the 1st study group

Responders		Nonresponders					
140 (53%)		124 (47%)					
		Null response		Partial response		Relapse	
		51 (41,1%)		34 (27,4%)		39 (31,5%)	
1st gt	2nd, 3rd gt	1st gt	2nd, 3rd gt	1st gt	2nd, 3rd gt	1st gt	2nd, 3rd gt
75 (40.5%)	65 (82.3%)	51 (27.6%)	0	28 (15.1%)	6 (7.6%)	31 (16.8%)	8 (10.1%)

In the first group patients, in total 30 various factors, influencing the treatment, are identified and analyzed:

1. The patient's factors (age, sex, the time from diagnosing hepatitis C till starting the therapy, co-morbidities, abdominal circumference, weight, BMI, blood count, ALAT, GGT, cholesterol, triglycerides, TSH, glucose level, insulin, insulin resistance, ANA, formation of neutralizing antibodies against alpha interferon, interleukin 28B gene polymorphism, a patient's compliance to therapy, harmful habits – smoking, alcohol consumption).

2. Viral factors (genotype, viral load).

3. Morphological changes (fibrosis stage, activity of inflammation).

2nd group – in order to determine IL 28B gene polymorphism in Latvia, there were selected 159 chronic VHC patients from total 299 under study, who:

✓ were the first from the queue included into the study. All second group patients were tested for interleukin 28B gene polymorphism in the 19th chromosome rs12979860 locus.

✓ 142 patients from this group, who had finished hepatitis C treatment, were determined and analyzed IL 28B polymorphism in relation to the therapy result. Patient characteristic is seen in Table 2.

Table 2.

Second group patients' characteristics

Factors	CC	Non-CC	All patients
Mean age, years	35	37	37 (18 – 68)
Number of patients, >40 years	15 (33%)	40 (42%)	54 (39%)
Males	27 (59%)	57 (59%)	84 (59%)
BMI, kg/m^2	25.2	26.2	25.9
BMI, >30kg/m^2	5 (11%)	12 (13%)	17 (12%)
1st genotype	21 (46%)	66 (69%)	87 (61%)
2nd ., 3rd genotype	25 (54%)	30 (31%)	55 (39%)
HCV-RNA, x10^6 IU/ml (1st genotype)	2.78	2.19	2.33
HCV-RNA, >600,000 IU/ml (1st genotype)	18 (39%)	47 (49%)	65 (46%)
ALAT, U/l	112 (17 – 325)	104 (22 – 447)	106 (17 – 447)
ALAT, >ULN	43 (93%)	85 (88%)	128 (90%)
GGT, U/l	46.8 (9 – 228)	88 (6 – 526)	75 (6-526)
GGT, >ULN	11 (24%)	40 (42%)	51 (36%)
Cholesterol, mM/l	4.14 (2.09 – 7.35)	4.6 (2.46 – 8.17)	4.48 (2.09 – 8.17)
Triglycerides, mM/l	1.17 (0.28 – 4.06)	1.17 (0.3 – 5.44)	1.11 (0.28 – 5.44)
Liver fibrosis* (*Knodell*)	0.975 (0 – 3)	1.2 (0 – 4)	1.13 (0 – 4)
F0	9 (21.9%)	21 (24.7%)	30 (23.8%)
F1	28 (68.3%)	47 (55.3%)	75 (59.5%)
F3	4 (9.7%)	12 (14%)	16 (12.7%)
F4	0	5 (5.9%)	5 (3.9%)
HAI index* (*Knodell*)	6.44 (1 – 12)	6.54 (2 – 13)	6.5 (1 – 13)
Steatosis* > 0 degree	34 (83%)	65 (76.5%)	99 (78.6%)
SVR	34 (74%)	50 (52%)	84 (59%)

* Missing data: histological examination n=11 (non-CC), n=5 (CC).

Material and methods

The research was confirmed by The Independent Ethics Committee for clinical investigation of drugs and pharmaceutical products performing its functions according to GCP and applicable regulatory requirements. The work was done in accordance with the international and LR laws and Helsinki declaration. Before undertaking the study, each patient got acquainted with the "Information to the patient" and gave a written consent for the participation in the study by signing "Statement of consent" and "Consent for data registration".

Most part of laboratory tests was done at LIC laboratory. Single tests were done at the laboratory of P.Stradins clinical university hospital (ANA), Genera genetics centre, Ltd. (IL 28B gene polymorphism) and P.Stradins clinical university hospital Department of Pathology (morphological examination of the liver tissue).

Chronic VHC diagnostics

In blood samples the following seromarkers were determined: anti-HCV and HCV-RNA, including HCV genotyping and identification of virus load (HCV in case of the 1st genotype).

For detection of anti-HCV in serum, ELISA tests by various companies were used (AxSYM system HCV version 3.0, Abbott, ASV; ORTHO HCV version 3.0, Ortho-Clinical Diagnostics Ltd., ASV; INNOTEST HCV Ab IV, Innogenetic, Belgium; MONOLISA Anti-HCV PLUS version 2, BIO-RAD, France).

For qualitative HCV-RNA detection in serum there were used commercially available reverse transcription polymerase chain reactions (PCR) method: Cobas AMPLICOR Hepatitis C Virus Test, v. 2.0, Roche Diagnostics, USA (sensitivity: >50 SU/ml, specificity: 100%).

HCV genotypes were determined using reverse hybridisation LiPA method (The VERSANT HCV Genotype Amplification Kit (LiPA), Bayer Corporation, Germany).

For quantitative HCV-RNA virus load detection there was used polymerase chain reaction: Cobas AmpliPrep/ Cobas TaqMan HCV test Roche, USA.

IL28B gene polymorphism detection

For testing IL28B gene rs12979860 polymorphism the standard molecular-biological methods were used in blood samples: classical DNA release from blood with phenolum, for amplification of polymerase chain reaction fragments, standard sequencing with Big Dye (Applied Biosystems). Genotypes were divided into CC, CT, TC, TT.

Detection of neutralizing antibodies against alpha interferon

For neutralizing antibody detection against alpha interferon there was used *iLite^{TM} antialpha assay* (BIOMONITOR, Ireland), in order to determine NABs in serum against human alpha interferon semiquantitatively, using lucipherase bioluminescence system.

Morphological examination

Morphological examination of the liver tissues was done at P.Stradins clinical university hospital Department of Pathology. For detection of inflammation activity and degree of fibrosis, Knodell's histological activity index was used.

Statistical analysis methods of results

The data statistical processing was done using the computer programmes SPSS v.15.0, MedCalc v12.0 and Microsoft Office Excel v.11. For the characteristics of patients' parameters the generally accepted descriptive statistical methods were used – summary tables with columns, bar graphs or histograms; indicators of central tendency and dispersion indicators – standard deviation (SD) and standard error (SE).

The meaning of parameter differences is estimated by 5% probability of statistical error, thus, if in the test results p-value was lesser or equal to 0.05, the differences between the study groups were recognized as statistically significant.

For the assessment of differences several statistical tests were used – if proportional data were conformed to the normal (Gaussian) distribution, for the quantitative difference analysis between several groups there was used the *analysis of variance (ANOVA)*, between two groups – *Student's t-test*. If the data were not conformed to the normal distribution, there was extra used a nonparametric *Mann-Whitney U test* for the comparison of two samples, or *Kruskal-Wallis H test* for the comparison or three and more samples. Conformity of proportional data to the normal distribution was determined by using *Kolmogorov-Smirnov test*.

Comparing the groups according to a certain qualitative parameter, Pearson's chi-squared (χ^2) or Fisher's exact criterion 2x2 tables were used. Considering χ^2 values and the number of freedom degrees (df), p value was stated.

In calculations *odds ratio* (OR) was used. It is the ratio of probability of favorable outcome to probability of unfavorable outcome. If OR>1, then probability of favorable outcome is greater than probability of unfavorable outcome, if 0<OR<1, then probability of unfavorable outcome is greater than probability of favorable outcome. Odds ratio was calculated, using the computer program MedCalc ver. 12.0 by formula (A x D) / (B x C), where:

A – patient rate from the study group (without effect) with specific exposure;

B – patient rate from the control group (with effect) with specific exposure;

C – patient rate from the study group (without effect) without specific exposure;

D – patient rate from the control group (with effect) without specific exposure.

In case any of values A, B, C, or D were zero, odds ratio was estimated according to a modified formula which is meant for small groups of numbers – [(2A + 1) x (2D + 1)] / [(2B + 1) x (2C + 1)]. Statistical significance was determined by Fisher's criterion. 95% confidence interval (95% CI) was calculated by the formula: 95% CI = ln OR ± 1.96.

To determine the correlation between variables, the correlation analysis was used. The calculation method of the correlation depended on the variable scale. If variables were calculated by the linear scale, then *Pearson's correlation coefficient* was used. If one of the variables has the ordinals scale, then nonparametric *Spearman's range correlation coefficient* was used.

In the current study the following interpretation of the correlation coefficient was used:

0 = neither correlation exists;

0 – 0.2 = very low correlation;

0.2 – 0.5 = low correlation;

0.5 – 0.7 = moderate correlation;

0.7 – 0.9 = high correlation;

0.9 – 1.0 = very high correlation.

In order to find out the possible impact of independent factors on the effectiveness of therapy, *binary logistic regression* was used.

Binary logistic regression

Since the dependent variable of the study *Therapy result* is binary, the *binary logistic regression* was used. Contrary to the ordinary linear regression, where by means of equation one can predict the outcome of the dependent variable, the aim of binary logistic regressions is to state the probability of the event, in this case – whether a patient, due to the effect of some factors, will occur in one, or in another group, whether he/she will not respond to therapy (0), or respond (1). Probability is ranging from 0 till 1, where the border is 0.5, if probability is <0.5, then the prognosis is good for the 1st group, if ≥ 0.5, then it is good for the second group. Probability was calculated by the equation: $p = 1/(1+e^{-z})$, where

$z = b_1x_1 + b_2x_2 + ... + b_nx_n + a$ (or the regression equation, x – values of independent variables, b – regression coefficients, a – regression constant).

e – mathematical constant (Euler's number) = 2.71828 (1828).

To acquire more precise results between the included independent variables there should not be any interrelations, therefore an extra correlation analysis for stating the correlation was performed.

Regression can have several methods of equation formations – *Enter, Forward* and *Backward*. All three were used. In the method *Enter* all independent variables are included in the equation, despite their impact strength on the dependent ones, thus the model is made by one step.

Methods:

✓ *Enter*

Regression model accepts only those patients where in the dependent variables there is no single missing variable. If there is the lack of at least one value, then the patient is excluded from the analysis.

R^2 value is calculated by two methods – Cox & Snell, which is used rarer, and Nagelkerke R^2, which is used more often. These indices show the influence of independent variables of the developed model on the dispersion of the dependent variable.

✓ *Backward Stepwise*

Using this method, by each step the one – the weakest independent variable is removed from the equation, while only the most significant independent variables remain in the equation.

✓ *Forward*

According to this method the indices of precision of this model were lower, therefore it was not further analyzed.

Results

Within the study 2 patient groups were analyzed.

1st group. To state the factors which affect the result of therapy, all treated patients were divided depending on the outcome of therapy – responders and nonresponders. The patient distribution is seen in Picture 3.

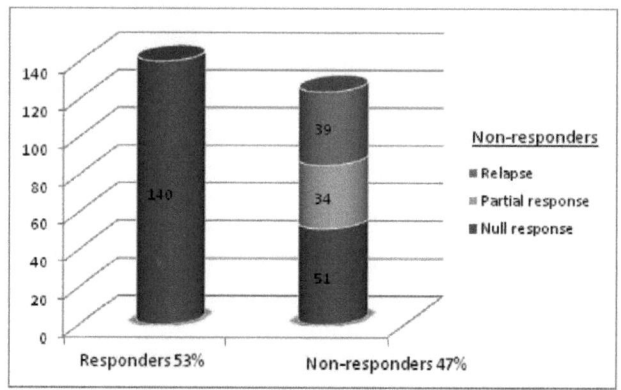

Picture 3. Patient distribution – responders/ nonresponders.

From all the included and treated chronic hepatitis C patients in the study – responders are 140 (53%), nonresponders – 124 (47%), who, as a result of therapy outcome are divided as follows: 51 patients were observed to have a null response – there is not achieved a hundredfold viral load reduction during 12 weeks, 34 patients were observed to have only a partial response – achieved at least a hundredfold HCV-RNA viral load reduction during 12 treatment weeks, but at the end of treatment HCV-RNA – positive, 39 patients – relapse – after treatment HCV-RNA negative, but 24 weeks after the end of treatment – positive.

Table 3.

Survey of results

Nr.	Parameters	Responders n=140, 53%	Nonresponders N=124, 47%	p
1.	Age, <45 years, %	58.6	41.4	0.005
	Age, ≥46 years	38.9	61.1	
2.	Body weight, kg	76.78	83.54	0.005
3.	BMI, kg/m^2	25.09	27.25	0.002
4.	GGT, U/l	36.0	63.5	0.000
5.	Insulin, μIU/ml	8.3	11.0	0.026
6.	IR, HOMA	1.78	2.51	0.031
7.	Fibrosis stage, *Knodell*	1.0	1.56	0.000
8.	HAI, *Knodell*	6.38	7.11	0.038
9.	Hemosiderosis, %	1.6	9.7	0.008
10.	HCV 1st genotype, %	40.5	59.5	0.000
	HCV 2nd, 3rd genotype, %	82.3	17.7	
11.	IL 28B CC genotype, %	89.7	10.3	0.001
	IL 28B non-CC genotype, %	59.8	40.2	

In both patient groups 30 factors influencing treatment result were analyzed. Statistically significant differences between responders and nonresponders patient groups were seen in 11 parameters (factors), see Table 3.

2nd group. Lately interleukin 28B coding gene polymorphism has been considered a significant influential factor on the treatment result, therefore patients of this group were determined IL 28B gene polymorphism and its effect on the therapeutic outcome.

Further on the most important factors in the results are analyzed separately.

Analysis of patient's factors

Age

All patients were divided into 2 groups according to the age – under 45 years and over 46 years. Further on there are summarized and analyzed the differences in different age groups in relation to the therapy outcome. The data on 263 patients were analyzed whose age was mentioned, 1 patient's age was not known at the moment of the data processing.

In the group under 45 years the patients responded to therapy more often (n=112, 58.6%), but in the group over 46 years – rarer (n=28, 38.9%), *p=0.005, Fisher's exact test* (Table 4.).

Table 4.

Differences by age groups

Age on starting therapy (< 45 >)		Therapy result		Total
		Non-responders	Responders	
0-45	N	79	112	191
	% Age on starting therapy	**41.4%**	**58.6%**	100.0%
	% Therapy result	**64.2%**	**80.0%**	72.6%
> 46	N	44	28	72
	% Age on starting therapy	**61.1%**	**38.9%**	100.0%
	% Therapy result	**35.8%**	**20.0%**	27.4%
Total	N	123	140	263
	% Age on starting therapy	46.8%	53.2%	100.0%
	% Therapy result	100.0%	100.0%	100.0%

Body weight

From all 264 patients included in the study, 181 patients (68.5%) were measured the body weight (the weight for 83 patients was not measured). The mean weight for analyzed patients was 78.87 (±15.21) kg. The mean weight differences in responders and nonresponders groups were analyzed.

Table 5.

The mean weight in responders/ nonresponders groups

Therapy result	Mean	Me-dian	Standard error	Standard deviation	Mini-mum	Maxi-mum	N
Non-responders	**83.54**	84.50	2.221	16.624	52	140	56
Responders	**76.78**	76.00	1.261	14.103	49	112	125
Total	78.87	78.00	1.130	15.208	49	140	181

In the group of responders there was diagnosed a lower body weight, on average 76.8 (±14.1) kg, in comparison to a nonresponders group, where it was on average 83.5 (±16.6) kg, the difference is statistically significant, *p= 0.005, Student's t-test* (Table 5.)

Body mass index (BMI)

From all 1st group patients, BMI was measured in 176 (67%) patients within the study. The mean BMI for the included patients was 25.75 (±4.36), which corresponds to the normal body weight. However, there are analyzed BMI differences between responders and nonresponders groups.

Table 6.

Differences of BMI in responders and nonresponders groups

Therapy result	Mean	Median	Standard error	Standard deviation	Mini-mum	Maxi-mum	N
Non-responders	**27.24654**	27.02641	.618274	4.543368	17.577	43.210	54
Responders	**25.09225**	24.18198	.374018	4.131162	17.998	38.104	122
Total	25.75322	25.07011	.328950	4.364011	17.577	43.210	176

In responders group there was observed a lower BMI, on average 25.09 (±4.13) kg/m^2 in comparison to nonresponders group where it is on average 27.25 (±4.54) kg/m^2, and the difference is statistically significant, *p=0.002, ANOVA* (Table 6.).

Gamma glutamiltranspeptidase

From all 264 patients included, 211 patients (80%) were determined GGT activity within the study. 110 patients (52.1%) within the study were found to have normal GGT activity, 101 patients (47.9%) – it was increased. Further on GGT activity data are analyzed in responders and nonresponders groups and the differences stated between groups.

During the study the differences were found in patients with normal or increased GGT activity. In the group with normal GGT activity 77 (70%) patients responded to therapy, while in the group of increased GGT activity – 36 (35.6%) patients, *p=0.000, Fisher's exact test* (Table 7.).

Table 7.

GGT differences in responders and nonresponders groups

GGT		Therapy result		Total
		Nonresponders	Responders	
Within normal range	n	33	77	110
	% GGT	30.0%	70.0%	100.0%
	% Therapy result	33.7%	68.1%	52.1%
Above the norm	N	65	36	101
	% GGT	64.4%	35.6%	100.0%
	% Therapy result	66.3%	31.9%	47.9%
Total	n	98	113	211
	% GGT	46.4%	53.6%	100.0%
	% Therapy result	100.0%	100.0%	100.0%

✓ GGT linear data

Table 8.

Mean GGT differences in responders and nonresponders groups

Therapy result	Mean	Median	Standard error	Standard deviation	Mini-mum	Maxi-mum	N
Nonresponders	113.4184	63.5000	12.18232	120.59884	6.00	797.00	98
Responders	55.2389	36.0000	6.09517	64.79256	8.00	526.00	113
Total	82.2607	51.0000	6.81610	99.00959	6.00	797.00	211

Statistically significant difference is observed also when analyzing the linear data. In the nonresponders group the mean GGT activity was higher (Me = 63.5 U/l) in comparison to the responders group (Me = 36.0 U/l), *p=0.000, Mann-Whitney U test* (Table 8.).

In the nonresponders group there was observed statistically significant difference between patients with a null response, partial response and relapse. At GGT activities within the normal range less patients (n=9, 27.3%) had null response and more – (n=17, 51.5%) relapse, in comparison to the patients' group in which GGT activity was higher. In this group a null response was found in 31 patients (47.7%), relapse – 16 patients (24.6%), *p=0.026, Pearson's chi-squared test* (Table 9.).

Table 9.

Differences in GGT activities in nonresponders group

GGT		Therapy result			Total
		Null response	Partial response	Relapse	
Within the normal range	N	9	7	17	33
	% GGT	27.3%	21.2%	51.5%	100.0%
	% Therapy result	22.5%	28.0%	51.5%	33.7%
Above the norm	N	31	18	16	65
	% GGT	47.7%	27.7%	24.6%	100.0%
	% Therapy result	77.5%	72.0%	48.5%	66.3%
Total	N	40	25	33	98
	% GGT	40.8%	25.5%	33.7%	100.0%
	% Therapy result	100.0%	100.0%	100.0%	100.0%

A similar tendency was observed, inspecting the patients' groups with various therapy response: in a null response group the patients were found to have a higher GGT activity more often (n=31, 77.5%) and rarer – normal GGT activity (n=9, 22.5%), in comparison to the relapse group, where an opposite tendency was seen – more often a normal GGT activity (n=17, 51.5%) and rarer – increased (n=16, 48.5%), *p=0.026, Pearson's chi-squared test* (Table 9.).

Insulin

From all 264 patients included, 191 patients (72.3%) within the study prior to starting the therapy were tested for the insulin level in blood. The mean insulin level in the patients under study was 9.5µIU/ml (median), which is within the normal range. Further on the data are calculated separately for responders and nonresponders groups in order to find the differences.

Table 10.

Mean insulin level in responders and nonresponders groups

Therapy result	Mean	Median	Standard error	Standard deviation	Mini- mum	Maxi- mum	N
Nonresponders	17.9200	**11.0000**	2.90048	21.51050	3.20	130.10	55
Responders	13.0404	**8.3000**	1.35731	15.82881	2.40	132.70	136
Total	14.4455	9.5000	1.28307	17.73233	2.40	132.70	191

Analyzing the insulin level in both patients' groups, a statistically significant difference was found. The mean insulin level in nonresponders group was higher – Me=11.0 µIU/ml, in comparison to the mean insulin level in the responders group Me=8.3 µIU/ml, *p=0.026, Mann-Whitney U test* (Table 10.).

Insulin resistance (HOMA)

Median insulin resistance parameter in patients included in the study was 2.05, which is within the normal range. The data are separately analyzed in the responders and nonresponders groups.

Table 11.

Insulin resistance parameter in responders and nonresponders groups

Therapy result	Mean	Median	Standard error	Standard deviation	Mini- mum	Maxi- mum	N
Nonresponders	7.0915	**2.5100**	2.39138	17.73498	0.66	107.20	55
Responders	3.5691	**1.7800**	0.52753	6.15200	0.50	50.20	136
Total	4.5834	2.0500	0.78880	10.90144	0.50	107.20	191

The differences between the groups were observed comparing the mean insulin resistance parameters. In the nonresponders group IR HOMA was 2.51, but in the responders group – 1.78, *p=0.031, Mann-Whitney U test* (Table 11.).

Within the study 3 patients had diabetes mellitus as a co-morbidity, from them 1 – responded to therapy, 2 – did not respond.

Hemosiderin

From all 1st group patients 237 (89.7%) within the study were done morphological examination and hemosiderin's presence was tested in the liver tissues. All in all, 13 patients were found to have hemosiderin during morphological liver tissue examination. Hemosiderin's presence is analyzed separately in responders and nonresponders groups.

Analyzing hemosiderin's presence in the liver tissues, the difference was observed in relation to the therapy effect. In the patients' group where hemosiderin was diagnosed in the liver tissues, proportionally a greater number of patients did not respond to therapy – 11 patients (84.6%), in comparison to the group where hemosiderin was not diagnosed – 102 patients (45,5%) did not respond to therapy. Besides, in the nonresponders group more often – 11 patients (9.7% cases) were diagnosed hemosiderin in the liver tissues in comparison to the responders group were it was observed only in 2 patients (1.6% cases), *p=0.008, Fisher's exact test* (Table 12.).

Table 12.

Differences of hemosiderin presence in responders/ nonresponders groups

Hemosiderin (qualitatively, is diagnosed/ not diagnosed)		Therapy result		In total
		Nonresponders	Responders	
Is diagnosed	N	11	2	13
	% HCV genotype	**84.6%**	**15.4%**	100.0%
	% Therapy result	**9.7%**	**1.6%**	5.5%
Not diagnosed	N	102	122	224
	% HCV genotype	**45.5%**	**54.5%**	100.0%
	% Therapy result	**90.3%**	**98.4%**	94.5%
In total	N	113	124	237
	% HCV genotype	47.7%	52.3%	100.0%
	% Therapy result	100.0%	100.0%	100.0%

Formation of neutralizing antibodies against alpha interferon

From all 1st group patients included, 121 were determined neutralizing antibodies against alpha interferon. 21 patients were diagnosed NABs prior to starting the therapy (a control group), 20 responders and 80 nonresponders VHC patients were tested for NABs after the end of treatment. Positive NABs was found in 5 patients (5%) from 100 after the end of the therapy – one patient (5%) from 20 in responders group and 4 patients (5%) from 80, who yielded a negative treatment result. In the nonresponders group 3 patients with diagnosed NABs received a full treatment course – 48 weeks and they showed good effect in the 12th therapy week. All 3 patients were seen to have a relapse after the end of treatment, 1 patient interrupted the treatment at the 12th week because no necessary viral load reduction was achieved – the therapy was considered to be ineffective – null response. Neither of the control group patients was seen to have positive NABs, Table 13.

Table 13.

Incidence of NABs in treated patients and control group

Determined NABs, n=121		
After therapy		Prior to therapy
Nonresponders, n=80	Responders, n=20	Control group, n=21
NABs, n=4 (5%)	NABs, n=1 (5%)	NABs, n=0

Other factors analyzed in the study

No statistically significant differences between responders and nonresponders groups were found analyzing the following patient's factors: patient's gender, smoking, alcohol consumption, skipped medicine doses, cholesterol and triglyceride level, ANA presence, US findings, presence of steatosis.

In total, 21 (7.9%) patients were found to skip the medicine dose, but not more than 10 times during the therapy course. Neither patient had skipped the medicine more than 10 times. However, statistically significant differences were not seen between responders and nonresponders groups due to the number of skipped medicine doses.

Within the study 232 patients (88%) were determined HBs antigen in serum. One patient was found a positive HBs result. This patient, as a result of the therapy, responded to therapy from hepatitis C virus infection.

Within the study 191 (72%) patients were done the test for HIV infection, all of them had negative result.

Importance of viral factors

HCV genotype

From all patients included into the study HCV 1st genotype was found in 185 (70.1%) patients, 2nd or 3rd genotype – 79 patients (29.9%) – 2nd genotype in 5 patients, 3rd genotype – 72 patients. Since the therapy in the 2nd and 3rd genotype cases is similar, and the number of the 2nd genotype patients is small, the results of these genotype patients are analyzed together. Further on there are analyzed HCV genotype differences in different patient groups.

Patients with HCV 2nd or 3rd genotype responded more often to therapy – 82.3% (65 patients), comparing to the 1st genotype patients who responded rarer to therapy – 40.5% (75 patients), $p=0.000$, Fisher's exact test (Table 14.).

Table 14.

HCV genotype differences in responders and nonresponders groups

HCV genotype		Therapy result		In total
		Nonresponders	Responders	
1st group (1st genotype)	n	110	75	185
	% HCV genotype	**59.5%**	**40.5%**	100.0%
	% Therapy result	**88.7%**	**53.6%**	70.1%
2nd group (2nd, 3rd genotype)	n	14	65	79
	% HCV genotype	**17.7%**	**82.3%**	100.0%
	% Therapy result	**11.3%**	**46.4%**	29.9%
In total	n	124	140	264
	% HCV genotype	47.0%	53.0%	100.0%
	% Therapy result	100.0%	100.0%	100.0%

No statistically significant differences were found, analyzing viral load parameters in responders and nonresponders groups.

Assessment of morphological changes of the liver tissue

Fibrosis

179 (68%) patients included in the study were found to have fibrosis – 126 patients were found to have fibrous, expanded portal fields (HAI = 1 point), 38 patients – bridging fibrosis (HAI = 3), 15 patients– cirrhosis (HAI = 4). 58 patients were not diagnosed fibrosis (HAI = 0). 27 patients lack the data on fibrosis. The higher is HAI index, the more progressing is hepatitis C virus induced inflammatory process in the liver. In order to analyze all the data and to be objective, the method for the data processing is chosen for linear data with normal distribution – Student's t-test.

Analyzing stage of fibrosis, it was found that in the responders group there is more common 0 (no fibrosis) and the 1st (fibrous, expanded portal fields) fibrosis stage, while in the nonresponders group more commonly was seen the 3rd (bridging fibrosis) and the 4th (cirrhosis) stage of fibrosis. In the responders groups fibrosis is seen in 90 (64.3%) patients, in the nonresponders group – 89 (72%) patients, however, statistically significant difference between these groups was not found.

Table 15.

Differences as to fibrosis stage in responders and nonresponders groups

Therapy result	Mean	Median	Standard error	Standard deviation	Mini-mum	Maxi-mum	N
Nonresponders	**1.56**	1.00	0.125	1.327	0	4	112
Responders	**1.00**	1.00	0.086	0.959	0	4	125
Total	1.27	1.00	0.077	1.179	0	4	237

If these data are analyzed by the linear method, one can find statistically significant difference between both groups. The mean indicator in the responders group is 1.0, but in the nonresponders group – 1.56, *p=0.000, ANOVA* (Table 15.).

Cirrhosis

Further degree of fibrosis is cirrhosis. Analyzing the incidence of cirrhosis in responders and nonresponders groups, one can find a statistically significant difference. In the responders group cirrhosis is seen in 3 (2.4%) patients, but in the nonresponders group – 12 (10.7%) patients, *p=0.014, Fisher's exact test*, while patients without cirrhosis respond more often (n=122, 55%), in comparison to cirrhosis patients who respond rarer (n=3, 20%), *p=0.014, Fisher's exact test* (Table 16.).

Table 16.

Presence of cirrhosis in responders and nonresponders groups

Presence of cirrhosis qualitatively (is present/ is not present)		Therapy result		Tota
		Nonresponders	Responders	
No cirrhosis	N	100	122	222
	% Presence of cirrhosis	**45.0%**	**55.0%**	100.0%
	% Therapy result	**89.3%**	**97.6%**	93.7%
Cirrhosis is present	N	12	3	15
	% Presence of cirrhosis	**80.0%**	**20.0%**	100.0%
	% Therapy result	**10.7%**	**2.4%**	6.3%
Total	N	112	125	237
	% Presence of cirrhosis	47.3%	52.7%	100.0%
	% Therapy result	100.0%	100.0%	100.0%

HAI index

27 patients lack morphological data and HAI index is not determined. For the rest of 237 patients the linear method was used for HAI index analysis and the mean HAI index was determined in responders and nonresponders groups.

Table 17.

Differences of HAI index in responders and nonresponders groups

Therapy result	Mean	Median	Standard error	Standard deviation	Mini-mum	Maxi-mum	N
Nonresponders	**7.11**	6.00	0.282	2.985	1	14	112
Responders	**6.38**	6.00	0.208	2.327	1	12	125
Total	6.73	6.00	0.174	2.677	1	14	237

In the study there were found HAI index differences in relation to the therapy effect. In the responders group the mean HAI index is 6.38, in the nonresponders group – 7.11, *p=0.038, ANOVA* (Table 17.).

Interleukin 28B gene polymorphism

From all hepatitis C patients included into the 2nd group of the study, who were determined IL 28B gene polymorphism, 53 patients (33%, 95% CI 25.7-40%) were found CC genotype, 84 patients (53%, 95% CI 45-61%) – CT (83 patients) or TC (1 patient) genotype and 22 patients (14%, 95% CI 8.6-20%) – TT genotype (Picture 4.).

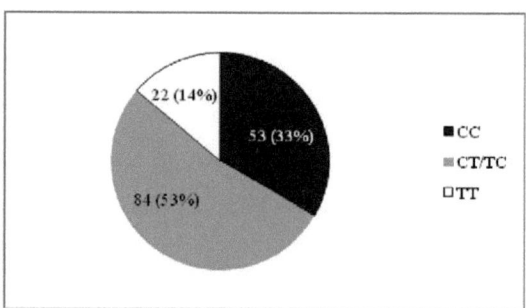

Picture 4. Interleukin 28B gene polymorphism

Further on there are analyzed the treatment results in 142 patients in relation to IL 28B gene polymorphism, to find out which IL 28B genotype is the most beneficial.

34 patients (73.9%) in CC genotype subgroup reached SVR (responders), in comparison to 50 patients (52.1%) in non-CC subgroup – 41 patients with CT/TC and 9 patients with TT, $p=0.002$, *Pearson's chi square test* (Table 18.).

Table 18.

Differences of therapy result in patients with various IL28B genotypes (CC, non-CC)

Therapy result		IL28B genotype		Total
		CC	Non-CC	
Nonresponders	N	4	35	39
	% IL28B	**8.7%**	**36.5%**	27.5%
Interrupted therapy /No result	N	8	11	19
	% IL28B	**17.4%**	**11.5%**	13.4%
Responded	N	34	50	84
	% IL28B	**73.9%**	**52.1%**	59.2%
Total	N	46	96	142
	% IL28B	100.0%	100.0%	100.0%

In CC subgroup 4 patients (8.7%) did not respond to therapy (all had relapse: 3 of them with HCV 1st genotype, 1 patient – with HCV 2nd genotype), comparing to 35 patients (36.5%), who did not respond to therapy in non-CC subgroup – 23 patients with CT/TC, and 12 patients with TT genotype (7 patients had a null response – all with HCV 1st genotype, 13 patients with partial response – 11 with HCV 1st genotype and 2 with HCV 3rd genotype, and 15 patients with relapse, all with HCV 1st genotype.

Table 19.

Differences of therapy result in HCV 1st genotype patients with various IL 28B gene polymorphism

			IL28B genotype		Total	p value
			CC	non-CC		
Therapy result	Nonresponders	n	3	33	36	
		% IL28B	15,79%	52,38%	43,90%	
HCV	Responders	n	16	30	46	**0.007367**
1st genotype		% IL28B	**84,21%**	47,62%	56,10%	
Total		n	19	63	82	
		% IL28B	100%	100%	100%	

It has already been proved earlier that, in relation to the therapy result, the most unfavorable one is HCV 1st genotype. The therapy result has been analyzed extra in relation to IL 28B gene polymorphism in HCV 1st genotype patients. Statistically significant difference was found between IL 28B genotype subgroups. In CC subgroup the patients with HCV 1st genotype responded to therapy more often – 16 patients (84.2%), in comparison to non-CC subgroup, where 30 patients (47.6%) underwent the treatment, *p=0.007, Fisher's exact test* (Table 19.).

Prognosis model of treatment result in chronic viral hepatitis C

While analyzing the differences, statistically significant differences were found ($p<0.05$) in 11 variables. These variables were selected for regression model as possible influential factors (independent variables), as well as HAI index, whose p-value is close to 5% border (Table 20.).

In the column „missing data" of Table 8.18. one can see what percentage of patients did not undergo this examination within the study. In this case from 264 patients 94 patients or 35.6% were chosen for the model from the total number of patients neither of whom had any missing variable.

Table 20.

Independent variables (factors possibly influencing therapy result)

Nr	Independent variable	P-value	Scale	Missing data (%)
1.	HCV genotype (1st – group 1; 2nd or 3rd – group 2)	0.000	Dichotomic variable	0.8%
2.	GGT	0.000	Lineary scale	20.1%
3.	IL28B genotype (1 – CC; 2 – non-CC)	0.001	Range scale	52.3%
4.	Body mass index	0.002	Lineary scale	33.3%
5.	Fibrosis	0.002	Range scale	10.2%
6.	Weight	0.005	Lineary scale	31.4%
7	Age group (1-<45 years; 2- >45 yrs.)	0.005	Dichotomic variable	0.4%
8.	Hemosiderin (1-is found; 2-not found)	0.008	Dichotomic variable	10.2%
9.	Presence of cirrhosis (1-no; 2-is)	0.014	Dichotomic variable	10.2%
10.	Insulin	0.026	Lineary scale	27.7%
11.	Insulin resistance HOMA	0.031	Lineary scale	27.7%
12.	HAI index	0.085	Range scale	10.2%

Since the calculation of the regression model and the structure differ from the classical difference analysis, including independent variables, then one can take also those parameters whose p value exceeds the classical 0.05, if it is close to it. Therefore also HAI index is included in the further calculations.

Odds ratio (OR) shows (Table 21.), how high is the prognosis not to respond to therapy at a certain independent variable.

Table 21.

Influence of independent variable to therapy result

Nr	Independent variable	Odds ratio (OR)	95% CI	P-value
1	HCV genotype 1st group	6.60	3.45 – 12.63	0.000
2	Hemosiderin is found	6.58	1.43 – 30.36	0.016
3	IL 28B genotype Non-CC	5.89	1.92 – 18.05	0.002
4	BMI extra weight and obesity	2.83	1.44 – 5.57	0.003
5	Cirrhosis is present	4.88	1.34 – 17.77	0.016
6	GGT is above the normal range	4.21	2.37 – 7.50	0.000

7	Age > 46 years	2.23	1.28 – 3.88	0.005
8	HAI index 8-12	1.60	0.95 – 2.69	0.078
9	Insulin is above the normal range	1.57	0.83 – 2.94	0.163
10	Insulin resistance HOMA above the normal range	168	0.89 – 3.15	0.109

By applying Spearman's correlation test, it was found that there exists a close relationship between insulin resistance HOMA and insulin (r_s=0.987, p=0.000), BMI and weight (r_s=0.859, p=0.000), as well as between HAI index, presence of cirrhosis and fibrosis (r_s=0.731, r_s=0.463, p=0.000), thus for the regression analysis there was left one significant or more precise variable from two in each pair (Table 22.).

Table 22.

Correlation analysis of independent variables

Spearman's correlation coefficient		Insulin (total)	Insulin resistance HOMA	Weight	BMI	HCV genotype 2	Hemosiderin	IL28B genotype	Age on starting therapy	GGT (total)	Fibrosis	Presence of cirrhosis
Insulin resistance HOMA	Correlation coefficient	.987										
	2-tailed significance (p-value)	.000										
	N	191										
Weight (dropped out)	Correlation coefficient	.238	.242									
	2-tailed significance (p-value)	.002	.001									
	N	174	174									
Body mass index	Correlation coefficient	.284	.296	.859								
	2-tailed significance (p-	000	.000	.000								

34

Spearman's correlation coefficient		Insulin (total)	Insulin resistance HOMA	Weight	BMI	HCV genotype 2	Hemosiderin	IL28B genotype	Age on starting therapy	GGT (total)	Fibrosis	Presence of cirrhosis
	value)											
	N	169	169	176								
HCV genotype 2	Correlation coefficient	-.004	-.003	-.120	-.203							
	2-tailed significance (p-value)	.957	.972	.108	.007							
	N	189	189	179	174							
Hemosiderin	Correlation coefficient	-.009	-.003	.035	.007	.161						
	2-tailed significance (p-value)	.905	.964	.659	.934	.014						
	N	173	173	163	160	235						
IL28B genotype	Correlation coefficient	.090	.097	.005	.075	-.242	-.022					
	2-tailed significance (p-value)	.321	.282	.959	.419	.006	.810					
	N	124	124	120	117	126	118					
Age on starting therapy (<45>)	Correlation coefficient	.172	.192	.023	.144	-.174	-.109	.024				
	2-tailed significance (p-value)	.017	.008	.758	.057	.005	.095	.792				
	N	190	190	180	175	261	236	126				

Spearman's correlation coefficient		Insulin (total)	Insulin resistance HOMA	Weight	BMI	HCV genotype 2	Hemosiderin	IL28B genotype	Age starting therapy	GGT (total)	Fibrosis	Presence of cirrhosis
GGT (total)	Correlation coefficient	.152	.160	.368	.354	-.140	-.198	.181	.122			
	2-tailed significance (p-value)	.057	.045	.000	.000	.043	.006	.059	.076			
	N	158	158	154	151	209	193	110	211			
Fibrosis (dropped out)	Correlation coefficient	.194	.201	.175	.180	-.047	-.078	.014	.382	.279		
	2-tailed significance (p-value)	.011	.008	.026	.024	.473	.236	.885	.000	.000		
	N	172	172	161	158	235	233	116	236	191		
Presence of cirrhosis (dropped out)	Correlation coefficient	.168	.155	.168	.160	-.096	-.133	.140	.294	.252	**.463**	
	2-tailed significance (p-value)	.028	.042	.033	.044	.142	.042	.135	.000	.000	**.000**	
	N	172	172	161	158	235	233	116	236	191	237	
HAI index	Correlation coefficient	.173	.188	.179	.233	-.025	-.066	-.030	.269	.254	**.731**	.285
	2-tailed significance (p-value)	.023	.013	.023	.003	.706	.314	.747	.000	.000	**.000**	.000
	N	172	172	161	158	235	233	116	236	191	237	237

To calculate the regression there are used 3 equation formation methods – *Enter, Forward* and *Backward*.

✓ *Enter* results

In the equation of the method *Enter* model are included all independent variables, despite the impact strength on the dependent, thus the model was made by one step.

This model takes only those patients where in independent variables there is not a single missing variable, in Table 8.18. with all the independent variables there are calculated the percentages of missing data. In this case 94 patients are taken from 264 patients or 35.6% from the total number of patients who do not have any missing variable.

Table 23.

Calculation of model coefficient *Omnibus* test

Steps		Chi-square	df	p value
Step 1	Step	28.356	8	**0.000**
	Block	28.356	8	**0.000**
	Model	28.356	8	**0.000**

Chi square table (Table 23.) shows whether the influence of independent variables of the step, block and model on the dependent variable is statistically significant.

Table 24.

Summary of model

Step	-2 Log possibility	Cox & Snell R^2 value	Nagelkerke R^2 value
1	86.145	0.260	**0.370**

Summary of model contains the information about R^2 values by two methods – Cox & Snell, which is used rarer, as well as Nagelkerke R^2, which is used more often. These parameters show part of the influence of the independent variables of the developed model on dispersion of the dependent variable. In this case these are 37%; it is the mean result (Table 24.).

Table 25.

Classification table for *Enter* model

Observed			Predicted		
			Therapy result		Correct prognosis
			Nonresponders	Responders	(%)
Step 1	Therapy result	Nonresponders	13	15	46.4 %
		Responders	8	58	87.9 %
total (%)					75.5 %

In the classification table (Table 25.) the information is surveyed on precision of regression and the proportion of correct prognosis is indicated – 75.5%. This table shows correctly predicted (grey color) and incorrectly predicted number of patients.

In the Table 26. variables in equation summarizes the information on influential variables and their significance.

Table 26.

Variables in equation for *Enter* model

Step 1	B	S.E.	Wald	df	Sig.	Exp(B)
Insulin resistance HOMA	-.039	.050	.610	1	.435	.961
BMI	-.118	.071	2.775	1	.096	.889
HCV genotype	**2.128**	**.858**	**6.146**	**1**	**.013**	**8.394**
Hemosiderin	-.058	1.523	.001	1	.969	.943
IL28B genotype	-1.106	.774	2.042	1	.153	.331
Age group	.004	.643	.000	1	.995	1.004
GGT	-.001	.003	.079	1	.779	.999
HAI index	-.196	.127	2.363	1	.124	.822
Constant	4.919	4.269	1.327	1	.249	136.832

The column B includes regression equation coefficients which depict each independent variable's effect on the dependent one.

SE – Standard error – shows the variability of B coefficient.

Wald – Wald's significance criterion: the higher it is, the intense is the impact of the independent variable on dependent variable.

Sig. – significance by Wald's criterion. It shows whether the influence of independent variable is statistically significant.

Exp(B) – coefficient e^B or OR (odds ratio) parameter.

Thus, judging by Table 8.24., the greatest influence is for variable HCV genotype, it is confirmed both by B coefficient, Sig, and Exp(B). The impact of the rest of the independent variables is not statistically significant.

According to this model the regression equation would look like this: $p = 1/(1 + e^{-z})$,

where z = HOMA × (-0.039) + BMI × (-0.118) + HCV genotype × 2.128 + Hemosiderin × (-0.058) + IL28B genotype × (-1.106) + age group× 0.004 + GGT × (-0.001) + HAI index × (-0.196) + 4.919.

For example, a patient with the following independent variables:

HOMA – 1.36, BMI – 24.032, HCV genotype – 2 (grupa), Hemosiderin – 2 (not found), IL28B – 2 (non-CC), age group – 1 (< 45 years), GGT – 54, HAI index – 5

z = 1.36 × (-0.039) + 24.032 × (-0.118) + 2 × 2.128 + 2 × (-0.058) + 2 × (-1.106) + 1 × 0.004 + 54 × (-0.001) + 5 × (-0.196) + 4.919 = 2.92818.

Inserting in the formula, $p = 1/(1 + e^{-2.92818}) = 1/(1 + 0.0534) = 1/1.0534 =$ **0.9493 or 94.93% possibility, that the patients will respond to therapy**.

✓ *Backward Stepwise* results

The model is formed by 6 steps – by each step the value of chi-square decreased, however, their changes are not statistically significant. Statistical significance of 6th model is very high, therefore this model can be practically useable.

Table 27.

6 steps of model

Step	-2 Log variability	Cox & Snell R^2	Nagelkerke R^2
1	86.145	.260	.370
2	86.145	.260	.370
3	86.147	.260	.370
4	86.226	.260	.369
5	86.696	.256	.364
6	89.125	.237	**.336**

R^2 parameter is slightly lower in comparison to the previous model – 0.336, however the difference is slight (Table 27.).

Table 28.

Classification table for *Backward* model

Observed			Predicted		Correct prognosis (%)
			Therapy result		
			Nonresponders	Responders	
Step 1	Therapy result	Nonresponders	13	15	46.4
		Responders	8	58	87.9
	Total (%)				75.5
Step 2	Therapy result	Nonresponders	13	15	46.4
		Responders	8	58	87.9
	Total (%)				75.5
Step 3	Therapy result	Nonresponders	13	15	46.4
		Responders	8	58	87.9
	Total (%)				75.5
Step 4	Therapy result	Nonresponders	13	15	46.4
		Responders	6	60	90.9
	Total (%)				77.7
Step 5	Therapy result	Nonresponders	13	15	46.4
		Responders	7	59	89.4
	Total (%)				76.6
Step 6	Therapy result	Nonresponders	**14**	**14**	50.0
		Responders	**6**	**60**	90.9
	Total (%)				**78.7**

Table 28. depicts each model's precision by steps. The highest precision – 79.7% is in the 6th step.

Table 29.

The variables in equation for *Backward* model

Steps		B	S.E.	Wald	Df	Sig.	Exp(B)
Step 1	Insulin resistance HOMA	-.039	.050	.610	1	.435	.961
	BMI	-.118	.071	2.775	1	.096	.889
	HCV genotype	2.128	.858	6.146	1	.013	8.394
	Hemosiderin	-.058	1.523	.001	1	.969	.943
	IL28B genotype	-1.106	.774	2.042	1	.153	.331
	Age group	.004	.643	.000	1	**.995**	1.004
	GGT	-.001	.003	.079	1	.779	.999
	HAI index	-.196	.127	2.363	1	.124	.822
	Constant	4.919	4.269	1.327	1	.249	136.832
Step 2	Insulin resistance HOMA	-.039	.050	.624	1	.429	.961
	BMI	-.118	.071	2.777	1	.096	889
	HCV genotype	2.127	.853	6.223	1	.013	8.389
	Hemosiderin	-.057	1.512	.001	1	**.970**	.944
	IL28B genotype	-1.106	.774	2.044	1	.153	.331
	GGT	-.001	.003	.079	1	.779	.999
	HAI index	-.195	.122	2.554	1	.110	.822
	Constant	4.920	4.264	1.332	1	.249	137.028
Step 3	Insulin resistance HOMA	-.039	.050	.622	1	.430	.962
	BMI	-.118	.071	2.785	1	.095	.889
	HCV genotype	2.125	.850	6.242	1	.012	8.370
	IL28B genotype	-1.104	.772	2.046	1	.153	.331
	GGT	-.001	.003	.079	1	**.779**	.999
	HAI index	-.196	.122	2.566	1	.109	.822
	Constant	4.802	2.909	2.725	1	.099	121.807
Step 4	Insulin resistance HOMA	-.039	.050	.596	1	**.440**	.962
	BMI	-.122	.069	3.067	1	.080	.885
	HCV genotype	2.154	.843	6.524	1	.011	8.620
	IL28B genotype	-1.142	.761	2.251	1	.133	.319
	HAI index	-.208	.115	3.298	1	.069	.812
	Constant	4.953	2.868	2.982	1	.084	141.576
Step 5	BMI	-.127	.068	3.492	1	.062	.880
	HCV genotype	2.056	.808	6.480	1	.011	7.817
	IL28B genotype	-1.113	.752	2.188	1	**.139**	.329
	HAI index	-.215	.114	3.557	1	.059	.807

	Constant	5.089	2.822	3.252	1	.071	162.259
Step 6	**BMI**	-.126	.067	3.569	1	**.059**	.882
	HCV genotype	2.377	.793	8.994	1	**.003**	10.774
	HAI index	-.191	.107	3.173	1	**.075**	.826
	Constant	2.502	2.094	1.428	1	.232	12.210

In the 6th step of the model only 3 variables left the regression – the most significant HCV genotype, BMI and HAI index. The last excluded variable is IL28B genotype, whose significance is 0.139. By increasing the selection border from 0.1 till 0.14, this variable remains in the equation, but then precision of the model decreases (Table 28., 29.).

Table 30.

Variables which are excluded from equation

			Significance	df	Significance
Step 2	Variables	**Age group**	.000	1	.995
	Total statistics			1	.995
Step 3	Variables	**Hemosiderin**	.001	1	.970
		Age group	.000	1	.998
	Total statistics			2	.999
Step 4	Variables	Hemosiderin	.001	1	.970
		Age group	.000	1	.989
		GGT	.079	1	.778
	Total statistics			3	.994
Step 5	Variables	**Insulin resistance HOMA**	.659	1	.417
		Hemosiderin	.001	1	.980
		Age group	.002	1	.963
		GGT	.060	1	.807
	Total statistics			4	.944
Step 6	Variables	Insulin resistance HOMA	.502	1	.479
		Hemosiderin	.017	1	.895
		IL28B genotype	2.316	1	.128
		Age group	.011	1	.915
		GGT	.281	1	.596
	Total statistics			5	.717

In Table 30. we can see the steps by which independent variables are removed from the model and equation. These are variables which in each model were of the least statistic significance – the lowest Wald's significance criterion in Table 8.27. (in column Wald).

According to this model the regression eaquation would look like this: $p = 1/(1 + e^{-z})$,

where $z = BMI \times (-0.126) + HCV\ genotype \times 2.377 + HAI\ index \times (-0.191) + 2.502$.

If we take the same patient with the following independent variables:

BMI – 24.032, HCV genotype – 2 (group 2), HAI index – 5

$$z = 24.032 \times (-0.126) + 2 \times 2.377 + 5 \times (-0.191) + 2.502 = 3.272968.$$

Inserting in the formula, $p = 1/(1 + e^{-3.272968}) = 1/(1 + 0.03789) = 1/1.03789$ = **0.9635 or 96.35% probability that the patient will respond to therapy.**

✓ *Forward* results

The model by this method *Forward* R^2 (0.296) and precision parameters (74.5%) were lower, therefore it is not analyzed further on. According to this model only two independent variables – HCV genotype and BMI were included in the regression equation.

✓ The method chosen: *Backward*

Taking into account results of all three models, one can most precisely prognosis hepatitis C treatment result by using the method *Backward*, in which 3 clinical parameters (independent variables) are taking into account – BMI, HAI index, HCV genotype. Precision of this model prognoses reach 78.7%. The formula can be placed into Excel file, thus easing the calculation of prognosis.

Table 31.

Prognosis model of hepatitis C response to therapy in Excel file

	BMI	1 – 1st gt. 2 – 2nd, 3rd gt. HCV genotype	HAI index
Multiply by coefficient B			
z-value			
z-value * -1			
e	2.718281828		
e^-z			
e^-z + 1			
Probability			

In Table 31. we can see the calculation formula in Excel file. In tinted table Windows are placed the patient's clinical parameters (independent variables) – BMI, HCV genotype and HAI index and acquire probability of response to therapy in percentage.

Table 32.

Probability of response to therapy for specific patient (1)

	BMI	1 – 1st gt. 2 – 2nd, 3rd gt. HCV genotype	HAI index
	24	2	7.11
Multiply by coefficient B	-3.024	4.754	-1.35801
z-value	2.87399		
z-value * -1	-2.87399		
e	2.718281828		
e^-z	0.056473149		
e^-z + 1	1.056473149		
Probability	**94.65%**		

Table 33.

Probability of response to therapy for specific patient (2)

	BMI	1 – 1st gt. 2 – 2nd, 3rd gt. HCV genotype	HAI index
	32	2	7.11
Multiply by coefficient B	-4.032	4.754	-1.35801
z-value	1.86599		
z-value * -1	-1.86599		
e	2.718281828		
e^-z	0.15474294		
e^-z + 1	1.15474294		
Probability	**86.60%**		

In Tables 32. and 33. we can see how probability of response to therapy is changing in HCV 3rd genotype patients with HAI 7.11 and BMI in the normal range, comparing it to obesity. Obese patient's probability of response to therapy decreases from 94.65% to 86.6%.

Table 34.

Probability of response to therapy for specific patient (3)

	BMI	1 – 1st gt. 2 – 2nd, 3rd gt. HCV genotype	HAI index
	24	1	7.11
Multiply by coefficient B	-3.024	2.377	-1.35801
z-value	0.49699		
z-value * -1	-0.49699		
e	2.718281828		
e^-z	0.60835907		
e^-z + 1	1.60835907		
Probability	**62.18%**		

Table 35.

Probability of response to therapy for specific patient (4)

	BMI	1 – 1st gt. 2 – 2nd, 3rd gt. HCV genotype	HAI index
	32	1	7.11
Multiply by coefficient B	-4.032	2.377	-1.35801
z-value	-0.51101		
z-value * -1	0.51101		
e	2.718281828		
e^-z	1.66697399		
e^-z + 1	2.66697399		
Probability	**37.50%**		

In Tables 34. and 35. we can see how probability of response to treatment changes in the patient with HCV 1st genotype and HAI index 7.11. If the patient is with normal BMI, the probability of his/her response to therapy is 62%, but in the obese patient the probability of response to therapy considerably decreases – up to 37.5%.

In Table 36. we can see that in an obese patient with HCV 1st genotype and considerable inflammation activity/fibrosis, the probability of response to therapy is slight – only 13.86%.

Table 36.

Probability of response to therapy for specific patient (5)

	BMI	1 – 1st gt. 2 – 2nd, 3rd gt. HCV genotype	HAI index
	32	1	14
Multiply by coefficient B	-4.032	2.377	-2.674
z-value	-1.827		
z-value * -1	1.827		
e	2.718281828		
e^-z	6.21521302		
e^-z + 1	7.21521302		
Probability	**13.86%**		

Table 37.

Probability of response to therapy for specific patient (6)

	BMI	1 – 1st gt. 2 – 2nd, 3rd gt. HCV genotype	HAI index
	24	1	2
Multiply by coefficient B	-3.024	2.377	-0.382
z-value	1.473		
z-value * -1	-1.473		
e	2.718281828		
e^-z	0.22923674		
e^-z + 1	1.22923674		
Probability	**81.35%**		

In Table 37. we can see that the patient with HCV 1st genotype, but normal BMI minimal inflammation activity (HAI = 2), probability for response to therapy is high – 81.35%. This result justifies to start the therapy even at slight changes in the liver not expecting when the disease progresses and the probability for treatment reduces.

Using this model, each specific patient is able to expect the possibility of response to therapy.

Conclusions

1. The patient's factors were found which affect the possibility of chronic C hepatitis response to therapy.

   1.1. Age – patients of younger age (under 45 years) responded to therapy more often (58.6%), comparing to much older patients (over 46 years) (38.9%).

   1.2. BMI – patients with normal BMI responded to therapy more often – 80.5%, comparing to patients with increased BMI (extra weight) – responded to therapy 61.5% or with a marked BMI – obesity – responded to therapy in only 52% of cases.

   1.3. Patients with a normal GGT activity responded to therapy more often – 70% cases, comparing to patients with increased GGT activity – in this patient group almost two times less patients 35.6% responded to therapy. In the patient group with increased GGT activity a zero response was observed more often, rarer – relapse, comparing to patients with normal GGT, where an opposite tendency was observed.

   1.4. In the responders group there was a lower mean insulin level (8.3) and the insulin resistance parameter (1.78), comparing to nonresponders group, 11.0 and 2.51 respectively.

   1.5. Presence of hemosiderin in the liver tissues was found comparatively rarely – 5.5% patients, while in nonresponders group it was seen more often (9.7%), comparing to responders (1.6%).

   1.6. Neutralizing antibodies against alpha interferon were found in 5% responders – similar in both groups (nonresponders and responders).

2. Viral factor, which affects the possibility of therapy, is the viral genotype – patients with HCV 2nd or 3rd genotype responded to therapy more often – up to 82%, comparing to patients with HCV 1st genotype, who responded to therapy on average in 40.5% cases.

3. Possibility of response to therapy also determines morphological changes in the liver tissues and the presence of cirrhosis:

    3.1. In the responders group there were lower mean parameters of fibrosis (1.0) and HAI index (6.38), comparing to nonresponders, 1.56 and 7.11 respectively.

    3.2. Cirrhosis patients responded to therapy rarer (20%), comparing to those chronic VHC patients, who did not have cirrhosis (55% responded to therapy).

4. In the current study in Latvia more commonly patients were found to have IL 28B gene CT genotype – 53% cases (n=84), CC genotype – 33% cases (n=53), most rarely – TT genotype of 14% patients (n=22). Patients with CC genotype responded to therapy more often – 74%, comparing to those with non-CC genotype subgroup, where 52.1% patients responded to therapy. HCV 1st genotype patients with IL 28B gene CC genotype responded to therapy up to 84%.

5. On the basis of 3 significant factors influencing the treatment (HCV genotype, BMI and HAI), it is possible to predict the possibility to respond to therapy for each patient by formula:

$$p = \frac{1}{1+e^{-z}}$$

z = BMI × (-0.126) + HCV genotype × 2.377 + HAI index × (-0.191) + 2.502.

HCV genotype:

1st genotype -1,

2nd, 3rd genotype -2.

Using this formula, prognosis for response to therapy can be calculated by 78.7% precision.

Practical recommendations

1. Prior to starting chronic hepatitis C treatment, one has to state the factors influencing the therapy result – BMI, virus genotype and HAI.

2. Considering the factors influencing the therapy result, one has to predict the possibility of SVR, using the developed model for chronic hepatitis C treatment prognosis.

3. In connection with the prognosis result, it is important to choose the individualized tactics:
   3.1. Prior to starting chronic hepatitis C therapy, one has to correct the factors which can be influenced (weight, BMI).
   3.2. To treat patients with slight HAI changes and normal BMI precociously.
   3.3. To consider the usefulness of the therapy for the 1st genotype patients with fibrosis/cirrhosis and obesity. To consider adding protease inhibitor to standard treatment.

4. All patients, attending the family doctor, should be examined for the possible viral hepatitis C (to determine anti-HCV), in order to diagnose the disease as early as possible. In a case of negative result, to repeat the examination every 5 years within one's lifetime.

References

1. Chen W, Wong T, Tomlinson G, *et al*. Prevalence and predictors of obesity among individuals with positive hepatitis C antibody in a tertiary referral clinic *J Hepatol* 2008;49(5):711-717.

2. Lavanchy D. The global burden of hepatitis C. *Liver Int* 2009;29:74–81

3. Heintges T, Wands JR. Hepatitis C Virus: Epidemiology and Transmission. Hepatology 1997;26(3):521-526.

4. Shepard CW, Finelli L, Alter MJ. Global epidemiology of hepatitis C virus infection. *Lancet Infect Dis* 2005;5:558–567.

5. European Association for the Study of the Liver. EASL Clinical Practice Guidelines: Management of hepatitis C virus infection. *J Hepatol* 2011;55:245–264

6. Tolmane I, Rozentale B, Keiss J, et al. Prevalence of viral hepatitis C in Latvia: a population based study. Medicina (Kaunas) 2011;47(10):532-535

7. Kau A, Vermehren J, Sarrazin C. Treatment predictors of a sustained virologic response in hepatitis B and C. *J Hepatol* 2008;49(4):634-651

8. Manns MP, McHutchison JG, Gordon SC, *et al*. Peginterferon alfa-2b plus ribavirin compared with interferon alfa-2b plus ribavirin for initial treatment of chronic hepatitis C: a randomized trial. *Lancet* 2001;358:958-965

9. Muir AJ, Bornstein JD, Killenberg PG, Atlantic Coast Hepatitis Treatment Group. Peginterferon alfa-2b and ribavirin for the treatment of chronic hepatitis C in blacks and non-Hispanic whites. *N Engl J Med* 2004;350:2265

10. Bonkovsky HL, Naishadham D, Lambrecht RW, *et al*. Roles of iron and HFE mutations on severity and response to therapy during retreatment of advanced chronic hepatitis C. *Gastroenterology* 2006;131:1440–1451

11. Berg T, von Wagner M, Nasser S, *et al*. Extended treatment duration for hepatitis C virus type 1: comparing 48 versus 72 weeks of peginterferon-alfa-2a plus ribavirisn. *Gastroenterol* 2006;130:1086-1097

12. Dai CY, Chuang WL, Ho CK, *et al.* Associations between hepatitis C viremia and low serum triglyceride and cholesterol levels: A community-based study. *J Hepatol* 2008;49(1):9-16

13. Khan KN, Yatsuhashi H. Effect of alcohol consumption on the progression of hepatitis C virus infection and risk of hepatocellular carcinoma in Japanese patients. *Alcohol* 2000;35:286-295

14. Mallat A, Hezode C, Lotersztajn S. Environmental factors as disease accelerators during chronic hepatitis C. *J Hepatol* 2008;48(4):657-665

15. Shiffman ML, Ghany MG, Morgan TR, *et al.* Impact of reducing peginterferon alfa-2a and ribavirin dose during retreatment in patients with chronic hepatitis C. *Gastroenterology* 2007;132:103

16. Bendtzen K, Ainsworth M, Steenholdt C, *et al.* Individual medicine in inflammatory bowel disease: Monitoring bioavailability, pharmacokinetics and immunogenicity of anti-tumour necrosis factor-alpha antibodies. *Scan J Gastroenterol* 2009;44: 774-781

17. Jēruma A. Hronisks vīrushepatīts C: bioķīmiskie un imūnģenētiskie diagnostiskie marķieri etioloģiskās terapijas efektivitātes prognozēšanai. Promocijas darbs. Rīga 2012

18. Kau A, Vermehren J, Sarrazin C. Treatment predictors of a sustained virologic response in hepatitis B and C. *J Hepatol* 2008; 49:634

19. Poynard T McHutchison J, Goodman Z, *et al.* Is an 'a la carte' combination interferon alfa-2b plus ribavirin regimen possible for the first line treatment in patients with chronic hepatitis C? The ALGOVIRC Project Group. *Hepatol* 2000;31:211-218

20. Everson GT, Hoefs JC, Seeff LB, *et al.* Impact of disease severity on outcome of antiviral therapy for chronic hepatitis C: lessons from the HALT-C trial. *Hepatology* 2006;44:1675–1684

21. Vīksna L. Vīrushepatīts C: norise, ārstēšana, prognoze, profilakse. Rīga: SIA Nacionālais apgāds, 2003. 26.-36.lpp.

22. Martinez-Bauer E, Forns X, Armelles M, et al. Hospital admission is a relevant source of hepatitis C virus acquisition in Spain. J Hepatol 2008;48(1):20-27.

23. Santantonio T, Wiegand J, Gerlach JT. Acute hepatitis C: current status and remaining challenges. *J Hepatol* 2008;49:625–633

24. Wiegand J, Deterding K, Cornberg M, *et al*. Treatment of acute hepatitis C: the success of monotherapy with (pegylated) interferon alpha. J Antimicrob Chemother 2008;62:860–865

25. Lettmeier B, Muhlberger N, Schwarzer R, et al. Market uptake of new antiviral drugs for the treatment of hepatitis C. *J Hepatol* 2008;49(4):528-536.

26. Di Bisceglie AM. Hepatitis C and hepatocellular carcinoma. *Hepatology* 1997; 26:34S.

27. Liang TJ, Rehermann B, Seeff LB, *et al*. Pathogenesis, natural history, treatment, and prevention of hepatitis C. *Ann Intern Med* 2000; 132:296.

28. Swain MG, Lai MY, Shiffman ML, *et al*. A sustained virologic response is durable in patients with chronic hepatitis C treated with peginterferon alfa-2a and ribavirin. *Gastroenterology* 2010;139:1593

29. Backus L, Boothroyd DB, Phillips BR, *et al*. Impact of sustained virologc response to pegylated interferon/ribavirin on all-cause mortality by HCV genotype in a large real-world cohort: The US Department of Veterans Affairs' experience. *Hepatology* 2010;52:428A

30. Deuffic-Burban S, Deltenre P, Louvet A, *et al*. Impact of viral eradication on mortality related to hepatitis C: amodeling approach in France. *J Hepatol* 2008;49:175–183

31. Afdhal NH. The natural history of hepatitis C. *Semin Liver Dis* 2004;24:3–8

32. Planas R, Ballesté B, Alvarez MA, *et al*. Natural history of decompensated hepatitis C virus-related cirrhosis. A study of 200 patients. *J Hepatol* 2004;40:823.

33. Thompson CJ, Rogers G, Hewson P, *et al*. Surveillance of cirrhosis for hepatocellular carcinoma: systematic review and economic analysis. *Health Technol Assess* 2007;11:1–206

34. Yang JD, Roberts LR. Hepatocellular carcinoma: a global view. *Nat Rev Gastroenterol Hepatol* 2010;7:448–458

35. Bartosch B, Thimme R, Blum HE, *et al.* Hepatitis C virus-induced hepatocarcinogenesis. *J Hepatol* 2009;51:810–820

36. O'Grady JO, Lake JR, Howdle PD. Comprehensive clinical hepatology. Mosby 2000. 6.1.-14. lpp.

37. Esteban JI, Sauleda S, Quer J. The changing epidemiology of hepatitis C virus infection in Europe. *J Hepatol* 2008;48:148–162.

38. Kamal SM, Nasser IA. Hepatitis C genotype 4: what we know and what we don't yet know. *Hepatology* 2008;47:1371–1383.

39. Rozentāle B. Hepatīts C Latvijā: Fakti un problēmas. Promocijas darbs. Rīga 1995.

40. Choo QL, Kuo G, Weiner AJ, *et al.* Isolation of a cDNA clone derived from a blood-borne non-A, non-B viral hepatitis genome. *Science* 1989;244:359.

41. Major ME, Feinstone SM. The molecular virology of hepatitis C. *Hepatology* 1997;25:1527.

42. Farci P, Alter HJ, Govindarajan S, *et al.* Lack of protective immunity against reinfection with hepatitis C virus. *Science* 1992;258:135.

43. Bonkovsky HL, Mehta S. Hepatitis C: a review and update. *J Am Acad Dermatol* 2001;44(2):159-182

44. Simmonds P. Variability of hepatitis C virus. *Hepatology* 1995;21:570.

45. Lau JY, Davis GL, Prescott LE, *et al.* Distribution of hepatitis C virus genotypes determined by line probe assay in patients with chronic hepatitis C seen at tertiary referral centers in the United States. Hepatitis Interventional Therapy Group. *Ann Intern Med* 1996;124:868.

46. Dusheiko G, Schmilovitz-Weiss H, Brown D, *et al.* Hepatitis C virus genotypes: an investigation of type-specific differences in geographic origin and disease. *Hepatology* 1994;19:13.

47. González-Peralta RP, Qian K, She JY, *et al.* Clinical implications of viral quasispecies heterogeneity in chronic hepatitis C. *J Med Virol* 1996;49:242.

48. Morgan TR, Ghany MG, Kim HY, *et al*. Outcome of sustained virological responders with histologically advanced chronic hepatitis C. *Hepatology* 2010;52:833

49. Alter MJ. Healthcare should not be a vehicle for transmission of hepatitis C virus. *J Hepatol* 2008;48(1):2-4.

50. Ciancio A, Manzini P, Castagno F, *et al*. Digestive endoscopy is not a major risk factor for transmitting hepatitis C virus. *Ann Intern Med*2005;142:903–909.

51. Wenzel RP, Edmond MB. Patient-to-patient transmission of hepatitis C virus. *Ann Intern Med*2005;142:940–941.

52. Siegel JD, Rhinehart E, Jackson M, Chiarello L, and the Healthcare Infection Control Practices Advisory Committee. 2007 Guideline for isolation precautions: preventing transmission of infectious agents in healthcare settings. Available from: http://www cdc gov/ncidod/dhqp/pdf/isolation2007, 12.02.2012.

53. Hauri AM, Armstrong GL, Hutin YJ. The global burden of disease attributable to contaminated injections given in health care settings. *Int J STD AIDS*2004;15:7–16.

54. Schreiber GB, Busch MP, Kleinmann SH, *et al*. The risk of transfusion-transmitted viral infections. *N Engl J Med* 1996;334:1685-1690.

55. Flora K, Schiele M, Benner K, *et al*. An outbreak of acute hepatitis C among recipients of intravenous immunoglobulin. *Ann Allergy Asthma Immunol* 1996;76:160-162

56. Healey CJ, Sabharwal NK, Daub J, *et al*. Outbreak of acute hepatitis C following the use of anti-hepatitis C virus-screened intravenous immunoglobulin therapy. *Gastroenterology* 1996;110:1120-1126

57. Yu MY, *Mason BL, Tanmkersley DL. Detection and characterization of hepatitisC virus RNA in immune globulines. Transfusion 1994;34:596-602*

58. Sīmanis R. Vīrushepatīts C hemofilijas slimniekiem: norise, ārstēšana, prognoze. Promocijas darbs. Rīga 2007.

59. Kurauchi O, Furui T, Itakura A, *et al.* Studies on transmission of hepatitis C virus from mother-to-child in the perinatal period. *Arch Gynecol Obstet* 1993; 253: 121–126

60. Silverman AL, Puccio JE, Kulesza GW, *et al.* HCV RNA is present in the menstrual blood of women with chronic hepatitis C infection. *Am J Gastroenterol* 1994; 89: 1201–1202

61. Silverman NS, Snyder M, Hodinka RL, *et al.* Detection of hepatitis C virus antibodies and specific hepatitis C virus ribonucleic acid sequences in cord bloods from a heterogeneous prenatal population. *Am J Obstet Gynecol* 1995; 173: 1396–1400

62. Moriya T, Sasaki F, Mizui M, *et al.* Transmission of hepatitis C virus from mothers to infants: its frequency and risk factors revisited. *Biomed Pharmacother* 1995; 49: 59–64

63. Paccagnini S, Principi N, Massironi E, *et al.* Perinatal transmission and manifestation of hepatitis C virus infection in a high risk population. *Pediatr Infect Dis J* 1995; 14: 195–199

64. Roudot-Thoraval F, Pawlotsky JM, Thiers V, *et al.* Lack of mother-to-infant transmission of hepatitis C virus in HIV-seronegative women: a prospective study with hepatitis C virus RNA testing. *Hepatology* 1993; 17: 772–777

65. Zanetti AR, Tanzi E, Paccagnini S, *et al.* Mother-to-infant transmission of hepatitis C virus. Lombardy Study Group on vertical HCV transmission. *Lancet* 1995; 345: 289–291

66. Lin HH, Kao JH, Hsu HY, *et al.* Absence of infection in breast-fed infants born to hepatitis C virus infected mothers. *J Pediatr* 1995; 126: 589–591

67. Kiyosawa K, Sodeyama T, Tanaka E, *et al.* Interrelationship of blood transfusion, Non-A, Non-B hepatitis and hepatocellular carcinoma: analysis by detection of antibody to hepatitis C virus. *Hepatology* 1990; 12: 671–675

68. Puro V, Petrosillo N, Ippolito G. Risk of hepatitis C seroconversion after occupational exposures in health care workers. *Am J Infect Control* 1995; 23: 273–277

69. Gordon SC, Patel AH, Kulesza GW, *et al.* Lack of evidence for the heterosexual transmission of hepatitis C. *Am J Gastroenterol* 1992; 87: 1849–1851

70. Soto B, Rodrigo L, Garcia-Bengoechea M, *et al.* Heterosexual transmission of hepatitis C virus and the possible role of coexistent human immunodeficiency virus infection in the index case. A multicentre study of 423 pairings. *J Intern Med* 1994; 236: 515–519

71. Fried MW, Shindo M, Fong T-S, *et al.* Absence of hepatitis C viral RNA from saliva and semen in patients with chronic hepatitis C. *Gastroenterology* 1992; 102: 1306–1308

72. Wang JT, Wang TH, Sheu JC, *et al.* Hepatitis C virus RNA in saliva of patients with posttransfusion hepatitis and low efficiency of transmission among spouses. *J Med Virol* 1992; 36: 28–31

73. Hyams KC, Phillips IA, Tejada A, *et al.* Three-year incidence study of retroviral and viral hepatitis transmission in a Peruvian prostitute population. *J Acquir Immune Defic Syndr* 1993; 6: 1353–1357

74. Lissen E, Alter HJ, Abad MA, *et al.* Hepatitis C virus infection among sexually promiscuous groups and the heterosexual partners of hepatitis C virus infected index cases. *Eur J Clin Microbiol Infect Dis* 1993; 12: 827–831

75. Woodfield DG, Harness M, Rix-Trott K. Hepatitis C virus infections in oral and injectable drug users. *N Z Med J* 1993; 106: 332–334

76. Mauser-Bunschoten EP, Bresters D, Van Drimmelen AA, *et al.* Hepatitis C infection and viremia in Dutch hemophilia patients. *J Med Virol* 1995; 45: 241–246

77. Troisi CL, Hollinger FB, Hoots WK, *et al.* A multicenter study of viral hepatitis in an United States hemophiliac population. *Blood* 1993: 81: 412–418

78. Wagner N, Rotthauwe HW. Hepatitis C contributes to liver disease in children and adolescents with hemophilia. *Klin Padiatr* 1994; 206: 40–44

79. Bukh J, Wantzin P, Krogsgaard K, *et al and* the Copenhagen Dialysis HCV Study Group. High prevalence of hepatitis C virus (HCV) RNA in dialysis

patients: failure of commercially available antibody tests to identify a significant number of patients with HCV infection. *J Infect Dis* 1993; 168: 1343–1348

80. Okuda K, Hayashi H, Kobayashi S, *et al.* Mode of hepatitis C infection not associated with blood transfusion among chronic hemodialysis patients. *J Hepatol* 1995; 23: 28–31

81. Gladziwa U, Schlipkoter U, Lorbeer B, *et al.* Prevalence of antibodies to hepatitis C virus in patients on peritoneal dialysis–a multicenter study. *Clin Nephrol* 1993; 40: 46–52

82. Ban BK, Yang CW, Yoon SA, *et al.* Prevalence and clinical course of hepatitis B and hepatitis C liver disease in ciclosporintreated renal allograft recipients. *Nephron* 1995; 70: 397–401

83. Ilako FM, McLigeyo SO, Riyat MS, *et al.* The prevalence of hepatitis C virus antibodies in renal patients, blood donors and patients with chronic liver disease in Kenya. *East Afr Med J* 1995; 72: 362–364

84. Coelho-Little M, Jeffers LJ, Bernstein DE, *et al.* Hepatitis C virus in alcoholic patients with and without clinically apparent liver disease. *Alcohol Clin Exp Res* 1995; 19: 1173–1176.

85. Zignego AL, Foschi M, Laffi G, *et al.* "Inapparent" hepatitis B virus infection and hepatitis C virus replication in alcoholic subjects with and without liver disease. *Hepatology* 1994; 19: 577–582

86. Oshita M, Hayashi N, Kasahara A, *et al.* Increased serum hepatitis C virus RNA levels among alcoholic patients with chronic hepatitis C. *Hepatology* 1994; 20: 1115–1120

87. Thein HH, Yi Q, Dore GJ, *et al.* Estimation of stage-specific fibrosis progression rates in chronic hepatitis C virus infection: a meta-analysis and meta-regression. *Hepatology* 2008; 48:418.

88. Tong MJ, el-Farra NS, Reikes AR, *et al.* Clinical outcomes after transfusion-associated hepatitis C. *N Engl J Med* 1995; 332:1463.

89. Takahashi M, Yamada G, Miyamoto R, *et al.* Natural course of chronic hepatitis C. *Am J Gastroenterol* 1993;88:240.

90. Yano M, Kumada H, Kage M, *et al.* The long-term pathological evolution of chronic hepatitis C. *Hepatology* 1996;23:1334.

91. Amin J, Law MG, Bartlett M, *et al.* Causes of death after diagnosis of hepatitis B or hepatitis C infection: a large community-based linkage study. *Lancet* 2006; 368:938.

92. Kenny-Walsh E. Clinical outcomes after hepatitis C infection from contaminated anti-D immune globulin. Irish Hepatology Research Group. *N Engl J Med* 1999;340:1228.

93. Powell EE, Edwards-Smith CJ, Hay JL, *et al.* Host genetic factors influence disease progression in chronic hepatitis C. *Hepatology* 2000;31:828.

94. Poynard T, Bedossa P, Opolon P. Natural history of liver fibrosis progression in patients with chronic hepatitis C. The OBSVIRC, METAVIR, CLINIVIR, and DOSVIRC groups. *Lancet* 1997;349:825.

95. Seeff LB. Natural history of hepatitis C. *Hepatology* 1997; 26:21S.

96. Marabita F, Aghemo A, De Nicola S, *et al.* Genetic variation in the interleukin-28B gene is not associated with fibrosis progression in patients with chronic hepatitis C and known date of infection. *Hepatology* 2011; 54:1127.

97. Vogt M, Lang T, Frösner G, *et al.* Prevalence and clinical outcome of hepatitis C infection in children who underwent cardiac surgery before the implementation of blood-donor screening. *N Engl J Med* 1999;341:866.

98. Hourigan LF, Macdonald GA, Purdie D, *et al.* Fibrosis in chronic hepatitis C correlates significantly with body mass index and steatosis. *Hepatology* 1999; 29:1215.

99. Clouston AD, Jonsson JR, Purdie DM, *et al.* Steatosis and chronic hepatitis C: analysis of fibrosis and stellate cell activation. *J Hepatol* 2001; 34:314.

100. Adinolfi LE, Gambardella M, Andreana A, *et al.* Steatosis accelerates the progression of liver damage of chronic hepatitis C patients and correlates with specific HCV genotype and visceral obesity. *Hepatology* 2001; 33:1358.

101.   Everhart JE, Lok AS, Kim HY, *et al.* Weight-related effects on disease progression in the hepatitis C antiviral long-term treatment against cirrhosis trial. *Gastroenterology* 2009; 137:549.

102.   Kallwitz ER, Layden-Almer J, Dhamija M, *et al.* Ethnicity and body mass index are associated with hepatitis C presentation and progression. *Clin Gastroenterol Hepatol* 2010; 8:72.

103.   Hézode C, Roudot-Thoraval F, Nguyen S, *et al.* Daily cannabis smoking as a risk factor for progression of fibrosis in chronic hepatitis C. *Hepatology* 2005; 42:63.

104.   Ishida JH, Peters MG, Jin C, *et al.* Influence of cannabis use on severity of hepatitis C disease. *Clin Gastroenterol Hepatol* 2008; 6:69.

105.   Hézode C, Zafrani ES, Roudot-Thoraval F, *et al.* Daily cannabis use: a novel risk factor of steatosis severity in patients with chronic hepatitis C. *Gastroenterology* 2008; 134:432.

106.   Freedman ND, Everhart JE, Lindsay KL, *et al.* Coffee intake is associated with lower rates of liver disease progression in chronic hepatitis C. *Hepatology* 2009; 50:1360.

107.   Modi AA, Feld JJ, Park Y, *et al.* Increased caffeine consumption is associated with reduced hepatic fibrosis. *Hepatology* 2010; 51:201.

108.   Ostapowicz G, Watson KJ, Locarnini SA, *et al.* Role of alcohol in the progression of liver disease caused by hepatitis C virus infection. *Hepatology* 1998; 27:1730.

109.   Pessione F, Degos F, Marcellin P, *et al.* Effect of alcohol consumption on serum hepatitis C virus RNA and histological lesions in chronic hepatitis C. *Hepatology* 1998; 27:1717.

110.   Oshita M, Hayashi N, Kasahara A, *et al.* Increased serum hepatitis C virus RNA levels among alcoholic patients with chronic hepatitis C. *Hepatology* 1994; 20:1115.

111.   Benvegnù L, Pontisso P, Cavalletto D, *et al*. Lack of correlation between hepatitis C virus genotypes and clinical course of hepatitis C virus-related cirrhosis. *Hepatology* 1997; 25:211.

112.   Roudot-Thoraval F, Bastie A, Pawlotsky JM, *et al*. Epidemiological factors affecting the severity of hepatitis C virus-related liver disease: a French survey of 6,664 patients. The Study Group for the Prevalence and the Epidemiology of Hepatitis C Virus. *Hepatology* 1997;26:485.

113.   Cacciola I, Pollicino T, Squadrito G, *et al*. Occult hepatitis B virus infection in patients with chronic hepatitis C liver disease. *N Engl J Med* 1999;341:22.

114.   Lambrecht RW, Sterling RK, Naishadham D, *et al*. Iron levels in hepatocytes and portal tract cells predict progression and outcomes of patients with advanced chronic hepatitis C. *Gastroenterology* 2011;140:1490.

115.   Fattovich G, Giustina G, Degos F, *et al*. Morbidity and mortality in compensated cirrhosis type C: a retrospective follow-up study of 384 patients. *Gastroenterology* 1997;112:463

116.   Hu KQ, Tong MJ. The long-term outcomes of patients with compensated hepatitis C virus-related cirrhosis and history of parenteral exposure in the United States. *Hepatology* 1999;29:1311

117.   García-Suárez J, Burgaleta C, Hernanz N, *et al*. HCV-associated thrombocytopenia: clinical characteristics and platelet response after recombinant alpha2b-interferon therapy. *Br J Haematol* 2000;110:98

118.   Adinolfi LE, Giordano MG, Andreana A, *et al*. Hepatic fibrosis plays a central role in the pathogenesis of thrombocytopenia in patients with chronic viral hepatitis. *BrJ Haematol* 2001;113:590

119.   Bruno S, Crosignani A, Maisonneuve P, *et al*. Hepatitis C virus genotype 1b as a major risk factor associated with hepatocellular carcinoma in patients with cirrhosis: a seventeen-year prospective cohort study. *Hepatology* 2007; 46:1350.

120.   Bartosch B, Thimme R, Blum HE, *et al.* Hepatitis C virus-induced hepatocarcinogenesis. *J Hepatol* 2009;51:810–820

121.   Ferri C, Sebastiani M, Giuggioli D, *et al.* Mixed cryoglobulinemia: demographic, clinical, and serologic features and survival in 231 patients. *Semin Arthritis Rheum* 2004;33:355

122.   Kompensējamo zāļu saraksts.

123.   Ng V, Saab S. Effects of a sustained virologic response on outcomes of patients with chronic hepatitis C. *Clin Gastroenterol Hepatol* 2011;9:923

124.   Russo MW. Antiviral therapy for hepatitis C is associated with improved clinical outcomes in patients with advanced fibrosis. *Expert Rev Gastroenterol Hepatol* 2010;4:535

125.   Cardoso AC, Moucari R, Figueiredo-Mendes C, *et al.* Impact of peginterferon and ribavirin therapy on hepatocellular carcinoma: incidence and survival in hepatitis C patients with advanced fibrosis. *J Hepatol* 2010;52:652

126.   Veldt BJ, Heathcote EJ, Wedemeyer H, *et al.* Sustained virologic response and clinical outcomes in patients with chronic hepatitis C and advanced fibrosis. *Ann Intern Med* 2007;147:677

127.   Calderon RM, Cubeddu LX, Goldberg RB, *et al.* Statins in the treatment of dyslipidemia in the presence of elevated liver aminotransferase levels: a therapeutic dilemma. *Mayo Clin Proc* 2010;85:349

128.   Onofrei MD, Butler KL, Fuke DC, *et al.* Safety of statin therapy in patients with preexisting liver disease. *Pharmacotherapy* 2008;28:522

129.   Advisory Committee on Immunization Practices. Recommended adult immunization schedule: United States, 2010. *Ann Intern Med* 2010;152:36

130.   Ghany MG, Strader DB, Thomas DL, *et al.* Diagnosis, management, and treatment of hepatitis C: an update. *Hepatology* 2009;49:1335

131. Bakerman S. Bakerman's ABC's of interpretive laboratory data. 4th ed. 255.-256.lpp.

132. Seeff LB, Everson GT, Morgan TR, *et al*. Complication rate of percutaneous liver biopsies among persons with advanced chronic liver disease in the HALT-C trial. *Clin Gastroent Hepatol* 2010;8:877-883

133. Tilg H. New insights into the mechanisms of interferon alfa: an immunoregulatory and anti-inflammatory cytokine. *Gastroenterology* 1997;112:1017.

134. Feld JJ, Hoofnagle JH. Mechanism of action of interferon and ribavirin in treatment of hepatitis C. *Nature* 2005;436:967

135. Tai AW, Chung RT. Treatment failure in hepatitis C: Mechanisms of non-response. *J Hepatol* 2009;50(2):412-420

136. Shiffman ML, Salvatore J, Hubbard S, *et al.* Treatment of chronic hepatitis C virus genotype 1 with peginterferon, ribavirin, and epoetin alpha. *Hepatology*2007;46:371–379

137. Manns MP, Wedemeyer H, Cornberg M. Treating viral hepatitis C: efficacy, side effects, and complications. *Gut* 2006;55:1350–1359

138. www.clinicaloptions.com/hep, 25.02.2012.

139. Sarrazin C, Susser S, Doehring A, *et al*. Importance of IL28B gene polymorphisms in hepatitis C virus genotype 2 and 3 infected patients. *J Hepatol* 2011;54:415–421

140. Fried MV, Shiffman ML, Reddy KR, *et al*. Peginterferon alfa-2a plus ribavirin for chronic hepatitis C virus infection. *N Engl J Med* 2002;347:975-982.

141. Conjeevaram HS, Fried MW, Jeffers LJ, *et al*. Peginterferon and ribavirin treatment in African American and Caucasian American patients with hepatitis C genotype 1. *Gastroenterology* 2006;131:470

142. Chen L, Borozan I, Feld J, *et al.* Hepatic gene expression discriminates responders and nonresponders in treatment of chronic hepatitis C viral infection. *Gastroenterology* 2005;128:1437–1444

143. Feld JJ, Nanda S, Huang Y, *et al.* Hepatic gene expression during treatment with peginterferon and ribavirin: identifying molecular pathways for treatment response. *Hepatology* 2007;46:1548–1563

144.   Sarasin-Filipowicz M, Oakeley EJ, Duong FH, *et al*. Interferon signaling and treatment outcome in chronic hepatitis C. *Proc Natl Acad Sci USA* 2008;105:7034–7039

145.   Gerotto M, Dal Pero F, Bortoletto G, *et al*. PKR gene expression and response to pegylated interferon plus ribavirin therapy in chronic hepatitis C. *Antivir Ther* 2004;9:763–770

146.   Taylor MW, Tsukahara T, Brodsky L, *et al*. Changes in gene expression during pegylated interferon and ribavirin therapy of chronic hepatitis C virus distinguish responders from nonresponders to antiviral therapy. *J Virol* 2007;81:3391–3401

147.   Distante S, Bjoro K, Hellum KB, *et al*. Raised serum ferritin predicts non-response to interferon and ribavirin treatment in patients with chronic hepatitis C infection. *Liver* 2002;22:269–275

148.   Lebray P, Zylberberg H, Hue S, *et al*. Influence of HFE gene polymorphism on the progression and treatment of chronic hepatitis C. *J Viral Hepat* 2004;11:175–182

149.   Thompson AJ, Muir AJ, Sulkowski MS, *et al*. Interleukin-28B polymorphism improves viral kinetics and is the strongest pretreatment predictor of sustained virologic response in genotype 1 hepatitis C virus. *Gastroenterology* 2010; 139:120-129

150.   Langhans B, Kupfer B, Braunschweiger I, *et al*. Interferon-lambda serum levels in hepatitis C. *J Hepatol* 2011;54(5):859-865

151.   Chen W, Wong T, Tomlinson G *etal*. Prevalence and predictors of obesity among individuals with positive hepatitis C antibody in a tertiary referral clinic. *J Hepatol* 2008;49(5):711-717

152.   Schmaling KB, Fiedelak JI, Bader J, *et al*. A longitudinal study of physical activity and body mass index among persons with unexplained chronic fatigue. *J Psychosom Res* 2005;58:375–381

153.   Angelopoulos N, Goula A, Tolis G. Current knowledge in the neurophysiologic modulation of obesity. *Metabolism* 2005;54:1202–1217

154.   Romero-Gomez M, Castellano-Megias VM, Grande L, Irles JA, Cruz M, Nogales MC, *et al.* Serum leptin levels correlate with hepatic steatosis in chronic hepatitis C. *Am J Gastroenterol* 2003;98:1135–1141

155.   Piche T, Vandenbos F, Abakar-Mahamat A, *et al.* The severity of liver fibrosis is associated with high leptin levels in chronic hepatitis C. *J Viral Hepat* 2004;11:91–96

156.   Shintani Y, Fujie H, Miyoshi H, *et al.* Hepatitis C virus infection and diabetes: direct involvement of the virus in the development of insulin resistance. *Gastroenterology* 2004;126:840–848

157.   Ortiz V, Berenguer M, Rayon JM, *et al.* Contribution of obesity to hepatitis C-related fibrosis progression. *Am J Gastroenterol* 2002;97:2408-2414

158.   Bressler BL, Guindi M, Tomlinson G, *et al.* High body mass index is an independent risk factor for nonresponse to antiviral treatment in chronic hepatitis C. *Hepatol* 2003;38:639-644

159.   Dentlere P, Louvet A, Lemoine M, *et al.* Impact of insulin resistance on sustained response in HCV patients treated with pegylated interferon and ribavirin: a meta-analysis. *J Hepatol* 2011;55(6):1187-1194

160.   Bernsmeier C, Duong FHT, Christen V, *et al.* Virus-induced over-expression of protein phosphatase 2A inhibits insulin signalling in chronic hepatitis C. *J Hepatol* 2008;49(3):429-440

161.   Vachon MLC, Factor SH, Branch AD, *et al.* Insulin resistance predicts re-treatment failure in an efficacy study of peginterferon-α-2a and ribavirin in HIV/HCV co-infected patients. *J Hepatol* 2011;54(1):41-47.

162.   Mehta SH, Brancati FL, Sulkowski MS, *et al.* Prevalence of type 2 diabetes mellitus among persons with hepatitis C infection in the United States. *Ann Intern Med* 2000;133(8):592-9

163.   El-Zayadi AR, Selim OE, Hamdy H, *et al.* Association of chronic hepatitis C infection and diabetes mellitus. *Trop Gastroenterol* 1998;19(4):141-4

164.   Aytug S, Reich D, Sapiro L, *et al*. Impaired IRS-1/PI3-kinase signaling in patients with HCV: a mechanism for increased prevalence of type 2 diabetes. *Hepatology* 2003;38(6);1384-92

165.   Masini M, Campani D, Boggi U, *et al*. Hepatitis C virus infection and human pancreatic beta-cell dysfunction. *Diabetes Care* 2005;28(4):940-1

166.   Anil KS, Raman BS. An intriguing relationship between type 2 diabetes mellitus and hepatitis C virus infection: the renal perspective. *Hepatitis Monthly* 2009;9(2):89-91

167.   Simo R, Harnandez C, Genesca J, *et al*. High prevalence of hepatitis C virus infection in diabetic patients. *Diabetes Care* 1996;19(9):998-1000

168.   Ozylkan E, Erbas T, Simsek H, *et al*. Increased prevalence of hepatitis C virus antibodies in patients with diabetes mellitus. *J Intern Med* 1994;235(3):283-4

169.   Sangiorgio L, Attardo T, Gangemi R, *et al*. Increased frequency of HCV and HBV infection in type 2 diabetic patients. *Diabetes Res Clin Pract* 2000;48(2):147-51

170.   Descamps-Latscha B, Jungers P, Witko-Sarsat V. Immune system dysregulation in uremia: role of oxidative stress. *Blood Purif* 2002:20(5):481-4

171.   Kalantar-Zadeh K, Ikizler T, Block G, *et al*. Malnutrition-inflammation complex syndrome in dialysis patients: causes and consequences. *Am J Kidney Dis* 2002;42(5):864-81

172.   Reddy KR, Shiffman ML, Rodriguez-Torres M, *et al*. Induction pegylated interferon alfa-2a and high dose ribavirin do not increase SVR in heavy patients with HCV genotype 1 and high viral loads. *Gastroenterology* 2010;139:1972

173.   Fried MW, Shiffman ML, Reddy KR, *et al*. Peginterferon alfa-2a plus ribavirin for chronic hepatitis C virus infection. *N Engl J Med* 2002;347:975–982

174.   Shiffman ML, Suter F, Bacon BR, *et al*. Peginterferon alfa-2a and ribavirin for 16 or 24 weeks in HCV genotype 2 or 3. *N Engl J Med* 2007;357:124–134

175.   Silva IS, Ferraz ML, Perez RM, *et al.* Role of gamma-glutamyl transferase activity in patients with chronic hepatitis C virus infection. *J Gastroenterol Hepatol* 2004;19:314–318

176.   Jorquera F, Monte MJ, Guerra J, *et al.* Usefulness of combined measurement of serum bile acids and ferritin as additional prognostic markers to predict failure to reach sustained response to antiviral treatment in chronic hepatitis C. *J Gastroenterol Hepatol* 2005;20:547–554

177.   Cobbold JFL, Patel JH, Goldin RD, *et al.* Hepatic lipid profiling in chronic hepatitis C: An *in vitro* and *in vivo* proton magnetic resonance spectroscopy study. *J Hepatol* 2010;52(1):16-24

178.   Bassedine MF, Sheridan DA, Felmlee DJ, *et al.* HCV and the hepatic lipid pathway as a potential treatment target. *J Hepatol* 2011;55(6):1428-1440

179.   Nkontchou G, Bastard JP, Ziol M, *et al.* Insulin resistance, serum leptin, and adiponectin levels and outcomes of viral hepatitis C cirrhosis. *J Hepatol* 2010;53(5):827-833

180.   Bhattacharya R, Shuhart MC. Hepatitis C and alcohol – interactions, outcomes, and implications. *J Clin Gastroenterol* 2003;36:242–252

181.   Pessione F, Degos F, Marcellin P, *et al.* Effect of alcohol consumption on serum hepatitis C virus RNA and histological lesions in chronic hepatitis C. *Hepatology*1998;27:1717–1722

182.   Poynard T, Bedossa P, Opolon P. Natural history of liver fibrosis progression in patients with chronic hepatitis C. *Lancet* 1997;349:825–832

183.   Mehta SH, Genberg BL, Astemborski J, *et al.* Limited uptake of hepatitis C treatment among injection drug users. *J Community Health* 2008;33:126–133

184.   Stoove MA, Gifford SM, Dore GJ. The impact of injecting drug use status on hepatitis C-related referral and treatment. *Drug Alcohol Depend* 2005;77:81–86

185.   Clark JM, Brancati FL, Diehl AM. The prevalence and etiology of elevated aminotransferase levels in the United States. *Am J Gastroenterol* 2003;98:960–967

186.   Inglesby TV, Rai R, Astemborski J, *et al.* A prospective, community-based evaluation of liver enzymes in individuals with hepatitis C after drug use. *Hepatology* 1999;29:590–596

187.   McCartney EM, Beard MR. Impact of alcohol on hepatitis C virus replication and interferon signaling. *World J Gastroenterol* 2010;16:1337–1343

188.   Seronello S, Ito C, Wakita T, *et al.* Ethanol enhances hepatitis C virus replication through lipid metabolism and elevated NADH/NAD+. *J Biol Chem* 2010;285:845–854

189.   Singal AK, Anand BS. Mechanisms of synergy between alcohol and hepatitis C virus. *J Clin Gastroenterol* 2007;41:761-772

190.   Hahn JA, Page-Shafer K, Ford J, *et al.*Traveling young injection drug users at high risk for acquisition and transmission of viral infections. *Drug Alcohol Depend* 2008;93:43–50

191.   Drumright LD, Hagan H, Thomas DL, *et al.* Predictors and effects of alcohol use on liver function among young HCV-infected injection drug users in a behavioral intervention. *J Hepatol* 2011;55(1):45-52

192.   Freedman ND, Curto TM, Lindsay KL, *et al.* Coffee consumption is associated with response to peginterferon and ribavirin therapy in patients with chronic hepatitis C. *Gastroenterology* 2011;140:1961

193.   McHutchison JG, Manns M, Patel K, Poynard T, *et al.* Adherence to combination therapy enhances sustained response in genotype-1-infected patients with chronic hepatitis C. *Gastroenterology* 2002;123:1061–1069

194.   McHutchison JG, Manns M, Patel K, *et al.*Adherence to combination therapy enhances sustained response in genotype-1-infected patients with chronic hepatitis C. *Gastroenterology* 2002;123:1061

195.   Benhamou Y, Bochet M, Di Martino V, *et al.* Liver fibrosis progression in human immunodeficiency virus and hepatitis C virus coinfected patients. The Multivirc Group. *Hepatology* 1999;30:1054–1058

196.   Czaja AJ, Carpenter HA, Santrach PJ, *et al.* Host- and disease-specific factors affecting steatosis in chronic hepatitis C. *J Hepatol* 1998;29:198–206

197.   Hui JM, Kench J, Farrell GC, *et al.* Genotype-specific mechanisms for hepatic steatosis in chronic hepatitis C infection. *J Gastroenterol Hepatol* 2002;17:873–881

198.   Poynard T, Ratziu V, McHutchison J, *et al.* Effect of treatment with peginterferon or interferon alfa-2b and ribavirin on steatosis in patients infected with hepatitis C. *Hepatology* 2003;38:75–85

199.   Adinolfi LE, Gambardella M, Andreana A, *et al.* Steatosis accelerates the progression of liver damage of chronic hepatitis C patients and correlates with specific HCV genotype and visceral obesity. *Hepatology* 2001;33:1358–1364

200.   Moriya K, Fujie H, Shintani Y, *et al.* The core protein of hepatitis C virus induces hepatocellular carcinoma in transgenic mice. *Nat Med* 1998;4:1065-1067

201.   Farinati F, Cardin R, De Maria N, *et al.* Iron storage, lipid peroxidation and glutathione turnover in chronic anti-HCV positive hepatitis. *J Hepatol* 1995;22:449-456

202.   Lee KS, Buck M, Houglum K, *et al.* Activation of hepatic stellate cells by TGF alpha and collagen type I is mediated by oxidative stress through c-myb expression. *J Clin Invest* 1995;96:2461-2468

203.   Paradis V, Mathurin P, Kollinger M, *et al.* In situ detection of lipid peroxidation in chronic hepatitis C: correlation with pathological features. *J Clin Pathol* 1997;50:401-406

204.   Antonelli G. Biological basis for a proper clinical application of alpha interferons. *New Microbiologica* 2008; 31:305-318

205.	Antonelli G, Gianelli G, Currenti M, *et al.*Antibodies to interferon (IFN) in hepatitis C patients relapsing while continuing recombinant IFN-α2 therapy. *Clin Exp Immunol* 1996;104:384-387

206.	Hou C, Chuang WL, Yu ML, *et al.* Incidence and associated factors of neutralizing anti-interferon antibodies among chronic hepatitis C patients treated with interferon in Taiwan. *Scan J Gastroenterol* 2000;12:1288-1293

207.	Zeuzem S, Fried MW, Reddy KR, *et al.* Improving the clinical relevance of pretreatment viral load as a predictor of sustained virological response (SVR) in patients infected with hepatitis C genotype 1 treated with peginterferon alfa-2a (40KD) (PEGASYS (R)) plus ribavirin (COPEGUS (R)). *Hepatology* 2006;44(Suppl. 1):267A–268A

208.	Salmeron J, Casado J, Rueda PM, *et al.* Quasispecies as predictive factor of rapid, early and sustained virological responses in chronic hepatitis C, genotype 1, treated with peginterferon-ribavirin. *J Clin Virol* 2008;41:264–269

209.	Farci P, Strazzera R, Alter HJ, *et al.* Early changes in hepatitis C viral quasispecies during interferon therapy predict the therapeutic outcome. *Proc Natl Acad Sci USA* 2002;99:3081–3086

210.	Moribe T, Hayashi N, Kanazawa Y, *et al.* Hepatitis C viral complexity detected by single-strand conformation polymorphism and response to interferon therapy. *Gastroenterology* 1995;108:789–795

211.	Enomoto N, Sakuma I, Asahina Y, *et al.* Mutations in the nonstructural protein 5A gene and response to interferon in patients with chronic hepatitis C virus 1b infection. *N Engl J Med* 1996;334:77–81

212.	Sarrazin C, Berg T, Lee JH, *et al.* Improved correlation between multiple mutations within the NS5A region and virological response in European patients chronically infected with hepatitis C virus type 1b undergoing combination therapy. *J Hepatol* 1999;30:1004–1013

213.	Pascu M, Martus P, Hohne M, *et al.* Sustained virological response in hepatitis C virus type 1b infected patients is predicted by the number of mutations within the NS5A-ISDR: a meta-analysis focused on geographical differences. *Gut* 2004;53:1345–1351

214.   Poynard T, Ratziu V, Charlotte F, *et al*. Rates and risk factors of liver fibrosis progression in patients with chronic hepatitis C. *J Hepatol* 2001;34:730–739

215.   Jacobson IM, Brown RS, Freilich B, *et al.* Peginterferon alfa-2b and weight-based or flat-dose ribavirin in chronic hepatitis C patients: a randomized trial. *Hepatology* 2007;46:971–981

216.   Knodell RG, et al. Formulation and Application of a Numerical Scoring System for Assessing Histological Activity in Asymptomatic Chronic Active Hepatitis. Hepatology 1981;1(5):431-435

217.   Бююль А, Цёфель П. SPSS: Искусство обработки информации. Анализ статистических данных и восстановление скрытых закономерностей: Пер. с нем. СПб. *ДиаСофтЮП*, 2005:257

218.   Manns MP, McHutchison JG, Gordon SC. Peginterferon alfa-2b plus ribavirin compared with interferon alfa-2b plus ribavirin for initial treatment of chronic hepatitis C: a randomized trial. *Lancet* 2001;358:958-965

219.   Hadziyannis SJ, Sette H Jr, Morgan TR. Peginterferon alfa-2a and ribavirin combination therapy in chronic hepatitis C: a randomized study of treatment duration and ribavirin dose. *Ann Intern Med* 2004;140:346-355

220.   Thompson AJ, Muir AJ, Sulkowski MS, *et al*. Interlaukin-28B polymorphism improves viral kinetics and is the strongest pretreatment predictor of sustained virological response in genotype 1 hepatitis C virus. *Gastroenterol* 2010;139:120-129

221.   Par A, Kisfali P, Melegh B, *et al*. Cytokine (IL-10, IL-28B and LT-A) gene polymorphisms in chronic hepatitis C virus infection. *Clin and Exp Med J* 2011;5(1):9-19

222.   Bacon BR, Gordon SC, Lawitz E, *et al*. Boceprevir for Previously Treated Chronic HCV Genotype 1 Infection. *N Engl J Med* 2011;364:1207-1217

223.   Zeuzem S, Andreone P, Pol S, *et al.* Telaprevir for retreatment of HCV infection. *N Engl J Med* 2011;364:2417-2428

224.   Thompson AJ, Fellay J, Patel K, *et al.* Variants in the ITPA gene protect against ribavirin-induced hemolytic anemia and decrease the need for ribavirin dose reduction *Gastroenterol* 2010:139(4):1181-1189

Publications on research theme

1. I.Tolmane, B.Rozentale, J.Keiss, F.Arsa, G.Brigis, A.Zvaigzne „Prevalence of Viral Hepatitis C in Latvia: Population Based Study" Medicina (Kaunas) 2011;47(10):532-535

2. I.Tolmane, B.Rozentāle, J.Keišs, L.Ivančenko, Z.Reinholde, N.Šubņikova, Ņ.Sumļaņinova, I.Kozlovska, S.Laivacuma, and R.Sīmanis „Interleukin 28B gene polimorphism and association with chronic hepatitis C therapy results in Latvia" *Hepatitis Research and Treatment* Volume 2012, Article ID 324090, 4 pages doi:10.1155/2012/324090, www.hindawi.com

3. I.Tolmane, B.Rozentale, J.Keiss, A.Ivanovs, R.Simanis „New toll to predict chronic hepatitis C treatment result for each patient" *Archieves Des Sciences* 2013, Vol 66, No 5:498-514

Acknowledgments

The author would like to express her thanks to her teacher in hepatology – professor Jazeps Keiss for support and encouragement in daily work. Great thanks to colleagues, who were rendering support in the process of planning and implementation of research work. The author felt indispensable inspiration and support in the working process from her family, great thanks to the dear ones for endurance and understanding.

Great thanks!

Financial support

Promotion thesis has been done under support of ESF project „Support to doctoral students for acquiring the study program and obtaining a scientific degree in Riga Stradins University", contract Nr. 2009/0147/1DP/1.1.2.1.2/09/IPIA/VIAA/009.

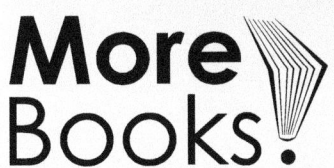
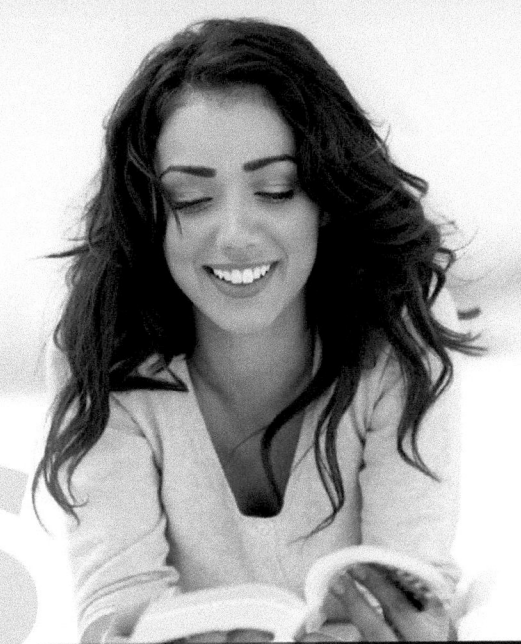
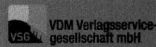

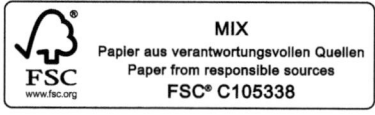